I0705034

LIVE EMPOWERED.

LEAD EMPOWERED.

HELPING YOU TAKE THE NEXT BEST STEP

AMIE TORKELSON

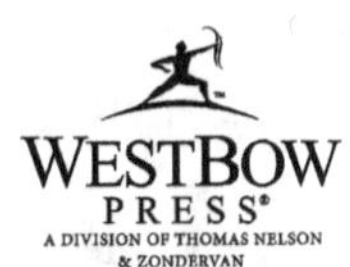

WESTBOW PRESS®
A DIVISION OF THOMAS NELSON
& ZONDERVAN

WestBow Press books may be ordered through booksellers or by contacting:

WestBow Press
A Division of Thomas Nelson & Zondervan
1663 Liberty Drive
Bloomington, IN 47403
www.westbowpress.com
844-714-3454

Because of the dynamic nature of the Internet, any web addresses or links contained in this book may have changed since publication and may no longer be valid. The views expressed in this work are solely those of the author and do not necessarily reflect the views of the publisher, and the publisher hereby disclaims any responsibility for them.

Any people depicted in stock imagery provided by Getty Images are models, and such images are being used for illustrative purposes only. Certain stock imagery © Getty Images.

Interior Image Credit: Hannah Sophia Photographer

Scripture quotations marked (NLT) are taken from the Holy Bible, New Living Translation, copyright ©1996, 2004, 2015 by Tyndale House Foundation. Used by permission of Tyndale House Publishers, a Division of Tyndale House Ministries, Carol Stream, Illinois 60188. All rights reserved.

ISBN: 979-8-3850-1845-1 (sc)
ISBN: 979-8-3850-1846-8 (hc)
ISBN: 979-8-3850-1844-4 (e)

Library of Congress Control Number: 2024902332

Print information available on the last page.

WestBow Press rev. date: 04/03/2024

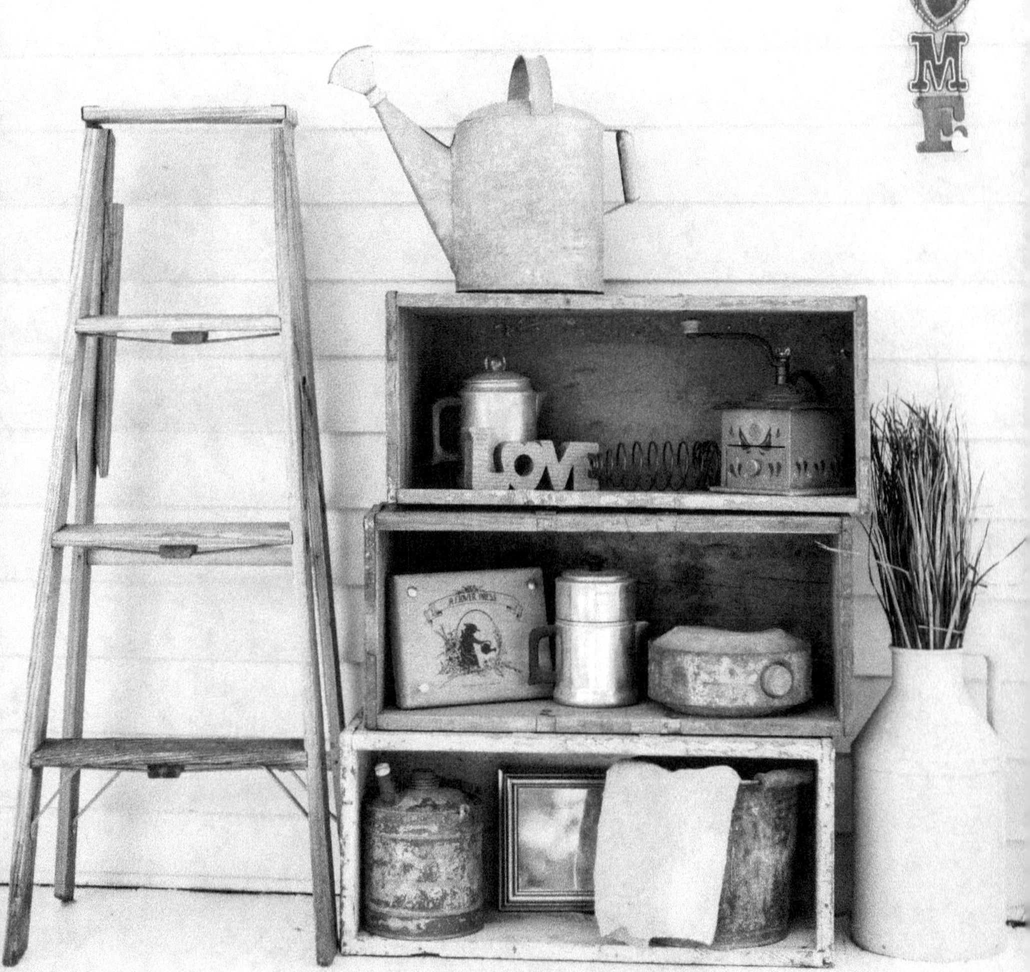

WELCOME
LOVE

This book is dedicated to all the people who have shared their dreams with me, whether you are walking them out or still dreaming. You have inspired me to share my passion for just starting right where you are. To those I know intimately and those I have yet to meet, here are the things I would tell my friends. I believe in you as much as I believe in them.

CONTENTS

INTRODUCTION

"He did this to humble you and test you for your own good. He did all this so you would never say to yourself, 'I have achieved this wealth with my own strength and energy.' Remember the LORD your God. He is the one who gives you power to be successful." (Deuteronomy 8:16–18).[1]

LIVE EMPOWERED

Are you living on purpose, for a purpose? Or are you of the thought that life is just happening and will keep happening whether you engage with it or not?

God has a big purpose for each one of us. He wants us to engage and make decisions that will impact and influence. Yet so many of us struggle to believe we are capable of, or even worthy of, achieving this great purpose for our lives.

We all have obstacles that hold us back: past wounds that need to be healed, our mental and physical health, the way we communicate with others, how we spend our days, and what we allow into our spaces. This book is all about the small steps you can take right now—just as you are in this moment—to live out your purpose.

Part of my inspiration for this book was the people in my life who I could see had such big potential but who hadn't quite found it in themselves. When they told me their dreams, I could look at them and say authentically, "That's incredible. You can do that!" The only problem was they couldn't believe it for themselves. It's what's inside of us, not what's outside of us, that holds us back from living our biggest dreams.

---

[1] Introduction
Deuteronomy 8:16–18 (New Living Translation).

I believed in these people so much, but I couldn't do the work for them. I know this because this is the journey I have gone through. I have had to go through my own process of healing and make the changes that allow me to live fully in my calling. I'm still growing and will be for my whole life.

Sometimes, it takes just one person who has walked the path before to encourage us to keep the course. I have had lots of people do that for me, and I hope to be one small voice that empowers you to do the work.

I am a firm believer in working through the garbage, not just pushing it down. When we try to push it down, it will always come back up. Someone gave me the visual of trying to hold a beach ball underwater. The farther down you push it, the higher it will pop into the air when it inevitably comes back up. The more we try to push down our emotions, the more out of control they will be when they finally burst. We have to work through our emotions for them to lose their power.

I want to hold your hand on this journey. You should get a few other people to do the same. I am so excited for you to be pursuing growth. It isn't about me giving you the answers. It is about reflecting and being introspective.

Everything you need is inside of you. Trust me, I know how ridiculous that can sound when you feel like you have nothing left, but I promise you there is hope and life on the other side. You don't have to be bound and limited by the negative beliefs that keep you stuck.

I want to give you practical tools to move forward, yes, but mostly, I want to be your cheerleader. I want to encourage you that no matter how hard it feels, keep leaning in.

Do the work. It will be worth it.

LEAD EMPOWERED

You, my friend, have something valuable to offer the world. You don't have to go learn a new skill. You don't have to go to school to become an expert. You don't need to be certified or qualified in the eyes of the world. Share what you already know. The truest thing you have to give is what is already inside of you.

Identify and speak truth to the lies that hold you back. Build the confidence to share your gift. If you are afraid to lead, it's not because you don't have something to share. You just need to identify what it is that's holding you back from sharing it.

This is the foundation of *Live Empowered. Lead Empowered.* When we live empowered, we live on purpose with a mission. We have something to share with others, and we propel them into motion, purpose, and passion. Here's the thing: a person doesn't have to have the same purpose and passion as you for you to inspire them. Creating a community with diverse strengths is actually more powerful and effective.

We all live with voices in our heads that try to hold us back. If we'd stop believing these lies, more people would be living their dreams and sharing their gifts. The spectrum of lies is wide and far. Sometimes we believe our knowledge is too basic or that it's common knowledge. Sometimes we believe no one will be interested in what we have to say.

The reality is that the thing that comes most easily to you is often the thing you should be sharing. That thing that is easy for you is hard for someone else, and what is easy for them might be hard for you. That is why we need each other. Think about that for a minute. You can use your knowledge to empower others. Just because something comes naturally to you doesn't mean you don't have the authority to share it. Our culture says if it isn't hard, it isn't valuable, but what if the fact that it comes easily to you actually makes it more valuable?

When you are living fully in your strength, people will be attracted to you even if other people have similar skills. Living confidently in your strength is magnetic.

FEEDING THE RIGHT WOLF

I ran year-round in high school. There was cross country in the fall, track in the spring, and off-season running in the winter and summer. I had the most invested coach in history. She wasn't just invested in our times and having a winning team. She was invested in us as people.

Every season, she would pick an animal as our theme. Throughout the season, she would share facts about the animal and relate them to us as a team and as runners. She always saw the temperature of the team: she could tell when we were down or struggling with our confidence. She used facts and stories about our chosen animal for the season to bring us together and encourage us.

One season, our animal was a wolf. This is when she introduced us to the tale of the two wolves. This story has appeared in many different forms and from many different sources over the years, but the heart of the story is a grandfather telling his grandson about a battle that happens within us. The battle is between two wolves: one that is evil and one that is good. The evil wolf is full of greed, jealousy, anger, and regret, and the good wolf is full of love, kindness, empathy, and generosity. The grandson asks which wolf will win. The grandfather replies that the wolf that wins will be the one you feed.

Why aren't more people living their dreams? Because they are feeding the wrong wolf.

This story illustrates so simply the heart behind the work that is to come in these pages. How can you feed the right wolf? It's a journey; it will shift little by little, not overnight. I am inviting you into these pages to look closer at which wolf you are feeding.

ENGAGING WITH YOUR STORY

The way to get the most out of these pages is by engaging with your story, so grab a journal or open your laptop and get ready to write. These pages are full of opportunities to engage with prompts and action steps because I believe it is so important to write things down. It raises your sense of commitment. After you set this book down, I don't want your inspiration to fade. I want these pages to hold you accountable and reinspire you every time you pick them up. The impact of these pages will be exponentially greater if you commit to taking concrete action steps.

I anticipate this journey will bring up a lot of feelings. Embrace them. Hold space for them. Take them to God. I challenge you to put aside all judgments of yourself, all thoughts of what others think of you, and all expectations for this journey. Be brave. Be willing to explore and process any emotions that come up without needing to have control of the process.

THE TIME IS NOW!

I am so excited for your journey. You are strong and brave, and I believe you can face that thing that has been on your "someday" list for years (and the reasons why it was on your "someday" list). You *can* do the thing you felt was too daunting, too big of a transition, or too out there.

I am all too familiar with the voices in my head—the ones hardest to silence or redirect—that tell me my vision is out of reach. They tell me my dream is too big, too wild, or can only happen far into the future. The voices try to convince me to give it up altogether. You just need one very important person to believe in you: you.

By the end of this book, you will have the direction, action steps, and motivation you need to start tackling the things that once felt out of reach. Actually, I hope you don't wait until the end! I hope you find the strength and inspiration to just begin. You don't have to get it all done next week, just keep pressing forward in the direction you want to go. You don't need to be fearless. You just need to be full of fight.

Rev. Robert H. Schuller asked the question, "What would you attempt to do if you knew you wouldn't fail?"[2] What does your mind run to? This question can reveal our deepest passion if we let the walls fall down.

Quick, get a pen. Start dreaming! What is your biggest passion? What about the world do you want to change? The thing that bothers us most is often the thing we are called to help change. Is it homelessness, slavery, addiction, poverty, or another humanitarian crisis? What gets you on your soapbox? What is your wildest dream? What would you like to impact? If you had no limitations and unlimited resources, what would you pursue?

No holdbacks.

---

[2] John Maxwell wrote, "My friend Robert Schuller once asked, 'What would you attempt to do if you knew you wouldn't fail?'" John C. Maxwell, *Sometimes You Win—Sometimes You Learn: Life's Greatest Lessons Are Gained from Our Losses* (New York: Center Street, 2013), 1.
Chapter 1

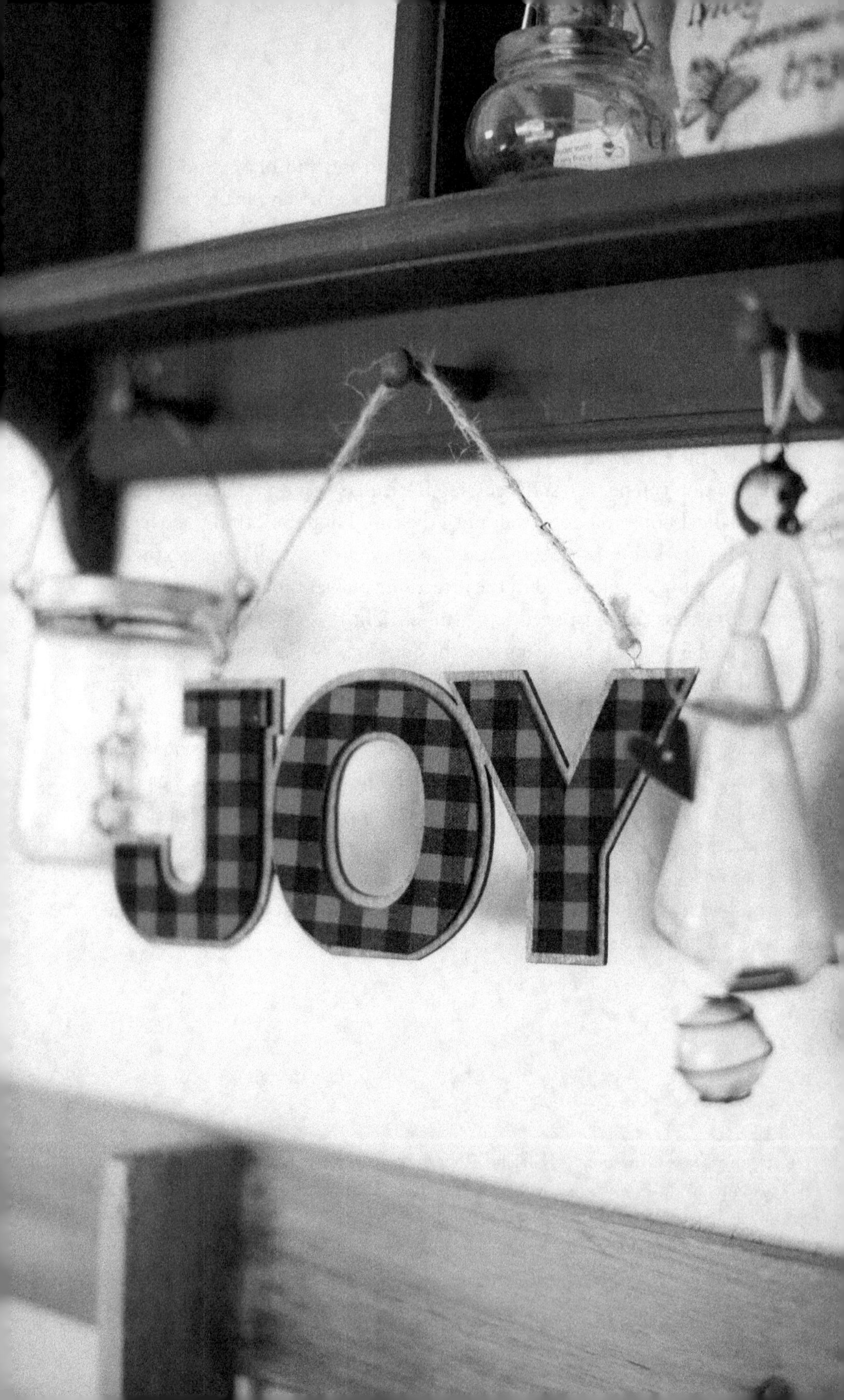

THE HEALING JOURNEY

1

WE ALL HAVE BAGGAGE

I so vividly remember one summer day when I was stuck in my home. The smoke from the forest fires was so thick it wasn't safe to go outside. I remember having a cup of tea and sitting with my toddler in the playroom. On this day, there wasn't anything I "should" be doing; there were conditions out of my control. I felt this wave of peacefulness. I wanted to do this every day just because I chose to, not because it was the only thing I could do.

This was a defining moment for me. It was a clear image of what my life *could* be like.

For so long, work was one of my biggest "drugs." It is so measurable. It is clear how much I have gotten done and how far there is to go before a project is complete. To be busy and to work was the way I proved my value. When I wasn't working, I was fighting massive battles with guilt and shame. The best way I found to relax was to move a hundred miles a minute. I know now that was coping, not relaxing.

Despite all this, I had a dream. My dream was to sit on the couch, drinking a cup of tea on a Saturday morning, just being present. I desperately wanted to enjoy a relaxing day with no agenda, to-do list, or guilt.

There would be days I set aside just to spend time with my family, but that's when the mental storms came. When I was spending time with my family, I would feel guilty for not working, but then I would start working and feel guilty for not spending time with my family. I so desperately wanted to break free from this cycle, but it felt impossible.

Then, in October 2019, God called me to a year of rest. At first, I couldn't imagine not working. I wanted to work. Work kept me feeling comfortable and safe.

And yet, just a month after I first heard that call, I committed to taking a year of rest.

That year of rest is why this book exists. I started writing as a way to process my feelings and take note of all the things I was learning.

I would not be where I am today in my healing journey if I hadn't made the decision to rest. It is the scariest thing I ever did, and I am so thankful I did it.

WHAT'S YOUR DRUG?

I was spending time with a friend who is a recovering alcoholic and fifteen years sober. She is someone who has turned their past into wisdom and insightfulness. During our conversation, she used the phrase "their drug of choice" in reference to a person who flipped cars. This phrase really struck me. She has known true addiction, and still, this is the phrase she used to describe what to many would seem like just a harmless hobby.

We often find it easy to identify an addiction when it is related to alcohol or drugs, but really, it's not about the substance or the activity. It is that we are using something to mask or run from our pain.

Bring awareness to what it is you are running to. Identifying what we are running to makes it so much easier to spot when we are running. From there, it is easier to find what we are running from.

For me, it has taken time to notice what I am running to because it is so subtle. This might be the same for you. One might eat a snack from their desk drawer or a piece of a chocolate bar, not giving any notice to what triggered their brain to want that snack or piece of chocolate. Okay, to be fair, when does chocolate not sound good? But bring awareness to it.

When I took my year of rest and put a hold on working, I started noticing more and more that food is another one of my drugs. Sugar and overeating are just other forms of stuffing and hiding.

Sugar is addictive. Dr. Mark Hyman, in his book *Eat Fat, Get Thin*, says, "Sugar and processed foods have been shown to be eight times more addictive than cocaine."[3] If you feed your body sugar every time it feels a bad emotion, you'll begin to crave it every time you feel bad. It's like Pavlov's dog experiment. At first, the dogs didn't respond to the sound of the bell they heard before they ate. They responded to the food. Once they learned to associate the bell with their food, they would salivate when they heard the bell. They expected food when they heard that sound.

If we have done an action long enough, we will automatically resort to that action even if it is hurting us.

I have found for myself that my food tendencies stem from childhood. I grew up with food insecurity. As an adult, I would scarf down food, overeat, and eat to feel secure. My weight didn't show it, but I've experienced all sorts of other health issues because of it. My body was telling me this overeating wasn't okay. It wasn't until I brought awareness to when I was eating that I started to unravel some of the emotions behind *why* I was eating.

The more aware you are of your "drug," the more you can choose healing over escape, and the more empowered you will become. You can choose to lean into the hard feelings rather than your drug. It could be anything, your phone, cigarettes, gambling, food, screen time, or so many other things. Something good can become bad if you are using it as your drug. Breaking these habits will be hard work, but it will be worth it to stop running.

One of the best things my naturopathic doctor has said to me is, "Embrace the turbulence." I have a type A personality. I am the kind of person who needs to have everything in order and under control, so this was hard to hear. I cried during that appointment. My doctor told me to ask for support. He gave weight to what a big transition it was for me to let go of food as my escape. He told me I was quitting a drug and was going through withdrawals.

Stick with it. Pray through it. Be brave.

God has a lot He wants to show us. Ultimately, He wants us to come to Him for healing. I have often found that when I am craving one of my "drugs," there is also a small voice inviting me to sit in the presence of God and talk with Him about my pain. Sometimes, I can be brave enough to

---

[3] Mark Hyman, *Eat Fat, Get Thin: Why the Fat We Eat Is the Key to Sustained Weight Loss and Vibrant Health* (New York: Little, Brown and Company, 2016), 190.

accept the invitation immediately. Sometimes, I fail and wish I would have listened and trusted. Either way, the invitation always stands.

This time may reveal what feels like an unbearable load. Give it to Jesus and create a support system. I have found time and time again when I am so frustrated and defeated, in tears, crying out to God, He is always there, but we have to pursue Him to hear from Him.

Matthew 7:7–8 says, "Keep on asking, and you will receive what you ask for. Keep on seeking, and you will find. Keep on knocking, and the door will be opened to you. For everyone who asks, receives. Everyone who seeks, finds. And to everyone who knocks, the door will be opened."[4]

None of these commands are passive. They all require our persistent effort.

EXPANDING YOUR CAPACITY FOR GOOD THINGS

I have noticed a pattern in my life: my worst days often follow my best days. When life is "too good," I self-sabotage. I had a moment a couple of months ago where this really struck me.

I was cleaning up the kitchen, and my husband was helping without me having to ask. Kennedy was playing so nicely. She came in to show us something and walked in on me and Dakota hugging. It was a perfect moment. After the kitchen was clean, Kennedy instructed me to sit with her at her fruit wash, and she made mounds of fake food for me to eat. This might sound like a small thing, but I struggled for a long time to be present while playing with my daughter.

This day was such a gift, and it didn't take long for my brain to catch up and try and take that gift away. I could—hear this—tell myself a lie to make a good feeling go away and not even notice. My brain would wander to all the mistakes I believed I had made that day. My mind would fill with worst-case scenarios and what-ifs. In an instant, I could go from feeling happiness and love to worry and dread.

This is a huge problem and is 100% a barrier to a joyful life. On that day, it was so clear to me that the life I was longing for still triggered a

---

[4] Matthew 7:7–8 (New Living Translation).

reaction in my brain. When I caught glimpses of it, I would sabotage it subconsciously. I have to bring my A game and fight against the lies my brain tells me when I'm having a good day.

This concept from *The Big Leap* has stuck with me: the author, Gay Hendricks, talks about recognizing when we are facing the limit of our personal struggle.[5] For example, if it is hard for you to receive love, the next time you notice yourself feeling loved, hold onto that feeling for as long as possible. Maybe it will only be for five seconds. That is okay. The next time, you may be able to hold onto it for eight seconds.

For me, it's not about how long you can hold onto the feeling. It's about bringing awareness to the good feeling and sitting with it. You need to hold it, welcome it, and allow it to stay. Hold onto love for as long as you can, and gradually your capacity to feel loved will grow. Eventually, you'll live your life feeling loved.

When I recognize I am believing a lie, I have two next steps I learned from one of my counselors to combat it:

1. I ask God to forgive me for believing this lie.
2. I ask God to show me the truth.

It is incredible how Jesus reveals His truth when you invite Him in. The change is more impactful when it comes from Jesus and not from my own strength and willpower. It has to come from surrender, not from force. There have been so many times in my life when the answer to my problem seemed so obvious, but it wasn't until I invited the power of the Holy Spirit that I truly heard the answer and it had a lasting impact. As long as I am fighting with willpower, I continue to fight the same battles over and over again. It isn't until I surrender to the truth Jesus has for me that my heart can receive it.

As I am changing what I believe about myself, I am expanding my capacity for good things. When I believe I am worthy of love, I can sit with the feeling of being loved. When I feel loved, I treat myself more lovingly. When I treat myself more lovingly, my capacity to receive love expands, creating more room to love and be loved. This is how we grow.

---

[5] Gay Hendricks, *The Big Leap: Conquer Your Hidden Fear and Take Life to the Next Level* (New York: HarperOne, 2009).

STAYING PRESENT

I mentioned earlier how I have struggled to be present with my daughter. It is something Jesus has been working on in me. For the first few years of her life, it was hard for me to spend five minutes with her before I self-sabotaged, grew tired, or went to do something "more productive."

This part of my story is still tender. When I imagined being a mom, I imagined having so much more to give. In a big way, my daughter was the catalyst for my growth.

Jesus has used my daughter to teach me how to be present. Part of me wishes I could have gone through the learning process in some other way. In an ideal life, I would have been able to give her undivided attention from the start, but really, I am so thankful it was my daughter who taught me this lesson. I hope my growth shows her that she was the thing in my life that meant enough. I hope she knows she was the catalyst that prompted me to do this work. I want her to grow up feeling more loved and worthy than if I'd had it together the whole time.

I am telling you this to encourage you because here's the thing: you have the choice to do the work. It isn't too late to change. As much as I wish I could have been more for my daughter sooner, that isn't an option now. What I can do is pray that Jesus will fill the gaps where I have failed as a human parent and that my daughter will feel abundantly loved despite my shortcomings. It's not about having it all together. It's about doing the work and letting those you love see you are still in process. I can pass these lessons on to my daughter by doing the work now.

John C. Maxwell advises us to use this as our motto:

> "I'm not where I'm supposed to be,
> I'm not what I want to be,
> But I'm not what I used to be.
> I haven't learned how to arrive;
> I've just learned how to keep on going."[6]

It's okay to let your loved ones see you on the journey.

---

[6] Maxwell, *Sometimes You Win—Sometimes You Learn*, 82.

LEARNED PATTERNS FROM CHILDHOOD

I grew up in a neighborhood that was close to a park and had lots of neighborhood kids. There were often group games of kickball or football. I enjoyed playing football most, but it seemed like almost every time we played, I would have to prove again to the boys that I was good enough to play.

Whoever the quarterback was wouldn't want to pass to me because I was a girl. I was often the only girl playing.

I could never throw a fit. I couldn't convince them with my words. I had to play hard to earn their approval. Once I started to play, they would see me catching passes, throwing, intercepting, and running just as well as the boys. The further we'd get into the game, the more they'd include me. By the end, I had as much playing time as any of the boys.

In a big way, this attitude has followed me into adulthood. I might not be the best, but I will work the hardest. This approach had many downfalls. For years, I looked outside of myself for validation. I needed someone to tell me I was good enough. I needed someone else to affirm my worth because I couldn't believe it for myself. I handed over my self-worth to whoever or whatever validated me. I wasn't succeeding out of fullness but out of emptiness.

When I formed relationships, I felt I had to earn the other person's approval and friendship. I had to perform. This left me vulnerable, and I would often be taken advantage of or manipulated. This would continue until the relationship became so toxic that it failed. I would do whatever they asked because I wanted to be irreplaceable.

This way of thinking caused me so much frustration and anger at my first job. Because of my high expectations for myself, I saw my coworkers as just doing the bare minimum. I felt like I was outperforming them but not being recognized for it. I would only feel valuable if I was recognized as valuable by others. If my coworkers didn't see me as irreplaceable, then I wanted to find somewhere where they would. Can you see the insecurity at play?

This is a call to take your blinders off. Go to someone you trust and ask them to help you find the toxic patterns in your life. This can feel so exposing and even painful, but it is so worth it. Start by talking to someone who knows you well and asking them these questions. Be open and consider what they have to say.

1. What do you think I seek most from other people? This could be love, attention, affection, affirmation, praise, compliments, etc.
2. Do you see any patterns in my relationships? For example, how do I typically make friends? Do I tend to attract people who are self-centered, pessimistic, depressed, angry, etc.? When might I cut off a friendship?
3. What do you think draws me to this type of person? What am I seeking, maybe even subconsciously, from them?

When you can identify what you are searching for in your relationships and find healthy ways to fill those needs, you will put your life on a whole new trajectory. You will live more wholly and find validation from within yourself.

Once you answer some of the questions above, brainstorm with a mentor, journal, pray, and meditate. Find out how God wants to fill those depleted places in a healthy way. Volunteering is a valuable place to begin. God designed us to serve others. There are so many benefits to giving our time, and it will fill our hearts in a genuine way.

You know the saying "You reap what you sow"? That means we have to sow what we want to reap. If we want positive things in our lives, it is our responsibility to put those positive things into motion. Pastor Ryan Oletzke talks about this concept in his sermon "Do Not Grow Weary." He says, "It's not if you're going to reap the consequence of your decisions. It's what you're going to reap . . . Sow the right actions and attitudes so we can reap a harvest of eternal life."[7]

HAS YOUR PAST SHAPED YOU?

I know people who think their childhood has little or nothing to do with who they are today. I know people who think it's best to just put their

---

[7] Pastor Ryan Oletzke, "Do Not Grow Weary," *True Hope Church*, September 5, 2021. Video, 49:04. https://www.truehopechurch.org/watch?sapurl=Lys0MWQ2 L3RlYWNoaW5ncy9taS8rNHg1ajI3eD9icmFuZGluZz10cnVlJmVtYmVkPXRyd WUmcmVjZW50Um91dGU9YXBwLndlYi1hcHAubGlicmFyeS5saXN0JnJlY2V udFJvdXRlU2x1Zz0lMkI0enEza3Y4.
Chapter 2

childhood behind them—they see no reason to let it affect their present. I also know people who are so stuck in their childhood it is like they are still there.

The best way to navigate your past is to find a balance between these extremes. I want to progress through my present forest of trials by using tools I acquired from my past.

Let's stay in the forest for a minute. In our adult journeys, we may find debris or fallen trees in our path. When we come across an obstacle, sometimes we must use the tools we were given in childhood to overcome them. Other times, we will find the tools useless or even counterproductive.

Too often, we hold onto the ineffective and frustrating tools from our childhood because they are the only ones we have, or at least the ones we are most comfortable with. We keep hitting the same obstacle with the same ineffective tools because we think we have no other choice. We want better tools but don't know how to make them or what to make. We become stuck behind the obstacle.

Then, someone spots us in the distance. They are more experienced than us—they've been down this road before. You're blocked by a barrier, so they can't physically reach you and give you their tool, but they climb up a limb so you can see them, and they can communicate with you. They begin explaining what to look for. They explain what to look for in the obstacle itself and point out the objects around you that you can transform into tools. They walk you through your frustration. They know it would be so much easier if they could toss you their tool belt, but that isn't an option. The best they can do is be patiently present while they walk you through how to make and maneuver the tool they know will work.

Finally, you get past the obstacle. You now have a new tool and more knowledge. The next time you face a fallen tree, you will have a little more confidence. You might instinctively reach for the ineffective tool first because it is so familiar, but soon you'll remember you have a new one now. It might take time to find your one good tool, but you will find it. Along your journey, you will meet more and more people who will help you make new tools and teach you how to use them. Before you know it, you will start getting rid of your ineffective tools because you no longer use them. You will soon find yourself sharing your new tools with other travelers.

Some people might start their adult journeys feeling like they are at a disadvantage. Maybe they don't have any tools in their tool belt, or the tools they do have are worse than not having any at all. That mindset will leave you stuck. No matter what we have experienced in childhood, it is our job as adults to search for the people effectively making their way through the forest and ask them for help. Sometimes, we will learn through our personal relationships. Sometimes, we will learn through books and teachings. The more tools we have, the more equipped we'll be to pursue and prepare better tools.

It is a journey. We won't just wake up with a new tool belt strapped to our hips. These tools can't be passed from one person to the next; they can only be replicated. Search for the people who have the tools you wish you had and start to replicate them.

In this forest of life, let's say your tool belt has to have five tools. The only way to get rid of the bad tools is to replace them with better ones. If you try to toss a bad one and don't replace it, the bad tool will just reappear.

As you continue to grow, what was once your best tool becomes your least used. You have found more effective tools. There will be a point where there is less transitioning of tools, but I don't think the process ever stops. Your tools will change with the seasons. There will always be more to learn and a better, more effective tool to reach for.

BE THE BEST YOU

So often, we default to comparing ourselves to our parents, but that comparison can hold us back. If your parents were 1,000 times bad and you're only trying to be better than them, you could still be 900 times bad. Whether you're settling for being better than your parents or striving to be better than your parents, it's still a distraction from the true goal: being the best version of ourselves.

I want to be the best Amie I can be—the best me I can be. I want to grow every day. I want to be strong and confident. I want to lead and be a positive influence. I want to be and do all God created me to be and do. If I am focused on being better than my parents, it means I am not focused on the big plans God has for me. I am looking down instead of up.

My friend said it in a way that made so much sense to me: "I realized the more I focus on not trying to be like my mom, the more I find myself being like her." We have to shift our focus from what we don't want to what we do want. When I find myself thinking I don't want to be, do, or become something, I stop myself and say the positive version of that thought out loud. Catch yourself. Claim the direction you want to go.

IT TAKES A TEAM

Our past has a way of showing up bigger and stronger when we are trying to move forward in life. This is especially true if we are trying to do something bold and impactful. Oftentimes it is a hint you are headed in the right direction. If we aren't careful, we can get tripped up by the baggage of our past. Progress is what will take away the power of our past.

Demystify and name your struggles. We can take away their power by unveiling the mystery and pressing into our pain. It can be scary as all get-out. I am not taking that away from you, but that's why you'll need to find a team of people to stand beside you and help you through the process. You can find this team through group counseling, a mentor, friends who you feel safe with, AA, or some other safe space.

Individual counseling—as opposed to group counseling—can also be extremely helpful. It is such an incredible feeling to sit with a professional and share something that is really scary to say out loud, something that feels so heavy it is hard to even say the words, and once the words are out, you can start to feel the weight of them dissipate. It wasn't too big after all.

I tend to keep things in my head because I fear being misunderstood. I worry I won't have the words to explain myself well. What if the person I'm talking to jumps to the wrong conclusion? What if I start to backpedal and defend myself, making it worse? I can get so wrapped up in worry I just shut down.

Misunderstood, guilty, shameful: these are the ugly feelings that come from not having a voice.

Find a safe place to do the work of healing. Find the people who make you feel safe. I do recommend working with trained professionals because even a split-second response from someone you are working with can be extremely discouraging. The wrong person can deflate or isolate instead of holding space and creating safety. Take the time you need to find the right team. There are a lot of great options out there.

My instinct has always been to do the hard things alone, but when I try to do them alone instead of alongside a gifted professional, facilitator, or guide, I end up digging myself into a deeper pit. I am still at a place in my healing journey where I need someone to affirm positive actions and thinking and help call out the false beliefs and lies. It is so beneficial to have someone further along in the journey to retrain your thinking and dig to your roots gracefully. Hiring a professional can just be a first step until you find those people in your daily life who can do the work with you.

A side note on finding a counselor: some people say it is like dating, and I agree. When you try a new counselor, it is like you are on a first date. You are getting to know whether they are the right fit for you. You are not stuck with the first counselor you try; it is okay to try a few. Ask the fundamental questions and see if their values align with yours. Someone who is a good fit for me may not be a good fit for someone else, but that doesn't mean they are a bad counselor.

Be picky. Don't try to force something that's not a good fit. You need to find someone who you can be completely open and vulnerable with.

It takes a team to embark on a healing journey. It takes hard work and vulnerability. In the end, it will all be worth it.

ACTION:

1. Do you know what your "drug" is? If you don't know, begin to notice what you reach for when you are uncomfortable. When do you find yourself escaping?

2. What are the most common lies you tell yourself? Keep a notepad with you. When you catch yourself in negative self-talk, write down what you can remember. These thoughts usually spiral pretty quickly, so it may take time to notice, but you will start catching these moments sooner and sooner. This is where you will begin your prayer of asking for forgiveness for believing these lies and having the truth revealed.

3. Combat the lies by writing the truths. Put them on your mirrors and door frames. Claim them daily.

4. Is it time to get a counselor? If the cost of counseling is a roadblock, look into programs like Celebrate Recovery, which is free and most often hosted at a church. Ask what your insurance covers. Look into local support groups. Call some churches or community centers and ask if they know of any local resources.

2

HEALING IS A JOURNEY

When you are building up a strong team of support around you, start looking for people who are ahead of you. Find the people who are where you would like to be and walk alongside them.

I love the saying, "Only take advice from people who have the results you want in life." Those results could be big or small, and that person doesn't have to be miles ahead of you—people only a few steps ahead can be immensely helpful.

I am always keeping an eye out for people to connect with. I might meet someone in a group setting or crossing paths at a yard sale. It begins with seeing a quality I admire and blossoms into having a role model to follow.

When I look for a mentor, I look for someone who has expertise in an area I would like to grow in but also lives a well-rounded life. I have different mentors with different knowledge and skill sets in different areas of life. I don't necessarily need to take health advice and business coaching from the same person.

I start by observing people. Do they lead a group? Do they serve in a ministry? I want to serve alongside them or volunteer to help. I identify the characteristics that drew me to them. I want to make sure the quality I was attracted to is consistent in their personality and aligns with their character as a whole.

Once I feel confident their character is authentic, I start asking questions. I ask them about the ways they do things and why they do it that way. I ask them how they got to where they are. One of my favorite questions to ask is what they are reading. This is a simple question that tells so much about a person. It shows where they are in their journey and where they are growing. It shows they are still pursuing their own growth.

Some people are natural-born leaders, and some aren't. Some people will naturally gravitate toward teaching, coaching, or mentoring, and for others, these skills won't come as naturally. This type of relationship might look different with different people. You can always learn from people who are pursuing their own growth.

Not everyone will make a good mentor. Some people offer lots of advice about things they have never done; this is a red flag. I have found that those who have knowledge about but no personal experience with a subject are often offering advice out of arrogance, pride, or insecurity.

I would rather work with a person who has experienced something firsthand than a person who has a lot of knowledge but has not taken the risk to try it. I would rather learn from the person who has started a business and had that business fail than the person who has read ten books about starting a business and never started. I am looking for someone who was brave enough to try and wise enough to evaluate and learn from what they did. I am looking for someone humble enough to see where they could have improved but proud enough to share their experience with confidence.

DRAWING HEALTHY BOUNDARIES WITH YOUR MENTOR

Having a mentor isn't always fun. The job of a mentor is to guide you through the hard stuff, which means sometimes they will tell you things you don't want to hear. You have to keep yourself accountable and not quit when your mentor tells you a hard truth. Remember, a mentor is someone you have given permission to speak into your life.

Be cautious about taking advice from only one person. I value having a handful of trusted voices who can cross-check the guidance I am receiving. Remember that your mentors are only human and will see things from only one perspective. They will have blind spots too.

Some people will be tempted to put their mentor in a decision-making role. Instead of seeking guidance and perspective from their mentor, they want their mentor to tell them what to do next. They feel paralyzed by decision-making and have no direction. I can empathize with this so much. This is an area I have struggled with in my own life. I went through a season of feeling so lost and wanting someone to just tell me what to do next.

A mentor can and should give perspective, but they should not make decisions for their mentee. The way I see it, mentorship is like counseling. A counselor doesn't just tell you the answers, even if they could skip you ahead five sessions by doing so. They know the importance of self-discovery. It is their job to guide you, not instruct you.

Be careful as a mentee that you don't pick a mentor who will make decisions for you. Pick one who will hold your hand and walk with you. There will be good people who love you and have good intentions but who will also want to make decisions for you. It is too painful for them to see others struggle, so they take on the burdens themselves. It's probably not intentional. They feel deeply and want to solve the problem, but that doesn't mean their methods will be helpful. Ultimately, I am not looking for someone to make decisions for me. I am looking for a handful of people who have been on the journey longer than I have and can share what they know.

In her book *Dare to Lead*, author Brené Brown suggests a tool called the "square squad." She says, "Get a one-inch by one-inch piece of paper and write down the names of the people whose opinions of you matter. It needs to be small because it forces you to edit."[8]

This practice works great for picking mentors. The names you write should be the names of people you know are going to be real with you. They won't shy away from telling you the truth, even when it is hard to hear. They will be trusted friends who don't do the work for you but walk alongside you.

I have found over and over that when I am longing for a mentor, and then I finally find "the one," I can esteem them too much. I put them on a pedestal so high I set them up for failure. This often begins from an innocent place of admiring their good qualities, but soon, I am shocked and disappointed when I find out they are real people with faults. Instead, I want to see them as humans with valuable wisdom to impart.

---

[8] Brené Brown, *Dare to Lead: Brave Work. Tough Conversations. Whole Hearts* (New York: Random House Large Print, 2018), 25.

No matter how much wisdom or maturity a person has, they are still human. When you put someone on a pedestal, you dehumanize them. They may feel like they aren't allowed to be flawed, or they would be failing you. In the past, I thought putting them on a pedestal was how I showed I respected them. Now I know this can be pressure that strains the relationship, causing it to wither, not flourish. We should expect imperfection, not be shattered by it.

Remember that you don't have to accept everything your mentor says. There is a beautiful balance between the willingness to learn and the confidence to challenge what you are told. This is an interesting dynamic for me; I want my mentors to feel respected. I don't want them throwing up their hands in frustration and wondering why they are helping someone who argues with everything they say. I believe a good mentor will give you their opinion and not be offended when you disagree with them. They will have confidence in your growth and won't need to control your journey. If you disagree with your mentor and they get mad, that to me is a red flag.

Having someone you can do life with, be real with, and let your walls down with is so worth the time and investment. It is a relationship, so it can be hard and messy sometimes, but the rewards will be greater than the struggles. To me, the value of having a mentor is having someone who has more perspective, knowledge, and experience than me. It's about working with someone who is passionate about helping others grow. The best mentors will not only be patient with your mistakes but will find reasons to be excited about them.

The best gift a mentor can offer is to accept us through our mistakes. The relationship shouldn't be about proving your worth or earning acceptance. A mentor should believe in you so much they are willing to invest their time and energy in you. And they won't need anything in return.

GRACE FOR THE JOURNEY

My life motto for years has been "We are all on a lifelong journey of growth." For years, I subconsciously thought I would complete my journey by the time I was thirty. If you are over thirty, you are probably laughing out loud right now.

When I was younger, people often commented about how mature I was. The first time I remember this happening was in sixth grade. I rode a bus that had both high school and middle school students. By the time I was in sixth grade, some of the other kids thought I was in high school. I always took that as a compliment.

I knew I had grown up fast. I was proud of that. Being seen as "beyond my years" was like a gold star. Responsibility was a role I both got pushed into and chose. I had more privileges and more obligations.

As I get older, I'm starting to see the setbacks of maturing early. In a way, I feel like I'm having to go back and mature in the areas I skipped. When I was a child, a seed was planted in my mind that I was further in life because I was seen as mature. So as an adult, I would often get frustrated with myself when I thought I should be further along in my healing journey. I thought I should be past the pain and moving on to better things. The irony is those thoughts only held me back more.

I love *Try Softer* by Aundi Kolber. It's a book that explains how in a world that is constantly telling us to try harder, we should actually "try softer." She wants us to slow down and look to God instead of forcing our way through our pain.[9] I was captivated by the way she spoke about her healing journey and progress. It gave me hope for what my future could look like. The problem was, when I first read the book, I took the message in the wrong direction to my default pattern of thought. I compared my progress to her progress. I longed to be on the other side of my journey.

As I said before, I have a type A personality. I like being able to check a box and consider a task complete. I sometimes find myself in a pile of stress when I think I'm taking too long to get something done. You know the old saying "An apple a day keeps the doctor away"? I once heard a joke that it doesn't have the same effect if you eat a week's worth of apples in one day. The point is any meaningful progress will be made little by little every day. When we rush the process, we end up with more problems than when we began.

It's no wonder we compare our stories to other people's. When we hear someone else's story, it sounds so picked up and neat. Somehow,

---

[9] Aundi Kolber, *Try Softer: A Fresh Approach to Move Us out of Anxiety, Stress, and Survival Mode—and into a Life of Connection and Joy* (Carol Stream: Tyndale House Publishers, 2020)

other people's mess sounds prettier than ours. We wonder why they are healed and we aren't. There's a reason for this. As a reader, you only see the messiness after it's been resolved—you get to see the beauty that came from the struggle. In your own story, the beauty is still being formed.

Believe that. Believe that beauty is being formed.

You have a beautiful story hidden in the mess. The word "posture" has been in my vocabulary a lot lately. It doesn't matter what we've gone through—what matters is the posture we hold our story in. That's what makes the story beautiful. I want to hold my story with open hands. I want to have a posture of restfulness, peace, grace, and kindness. I am in progress, but this is what I am striving for.

Books like *Try Softer* illuminate just how damaging it is to be hard on yourself. I can try to put it in a certain light and convince myself it's not "that bad" to be hard on yourself. When you compare it to loving yourself, you see just how harmful it is.

When I stopped rushing through the pain and started moving through the pain, it changed my entire healing journey. Moving through the pain means being gentle with myself. It means loving myself through the pain, not judging myself or trying to conquer the pain. My wiring tells me to fight and conquer. I have an inner football coach who demands I push harder, run faster, and keep going. What I need is to foster my inner yoga instructor. She says, "Listen to your body. You should feel the stretch, but it shouldn't be painful."

It is okay to be in progress. It is okay if that progress is messy. This is for me to hear as much as you. Moving through the pain with love and kindness for yourself will actually get you farther faster than forcing and pushing through the journey.

Moving through the pain looks like opening the door to it and inviting it in for tea. It looks like sitting on the couch with your pain and letting it tell you how it feels. You can't try to cut the time short or run out the back door. Moving through the pain is letting it know it is welcome at any time.

I used to be proud of the fact that I hadn't cried in years. I was so disconnected from my pain for so long in my teen years. It was my way of coping. I literally did not know how to let my guard down. Now I feel sad for that girl. I see now that this all shows just how much pain I was in.

Years later, I found myself unraveling. I was desperately trying to work through the pain, and it felt monstrous. It felt unbearable. This is the phase where I was pushing through. I treated my heart like it was a factory item passing inspection. I wanted it to pass with flying colors and move on.

The feelings are scary when they are on our doorstep. How was I supposed to invite them in? I wanted to manage them while they were out there and not let them get too close. For years, I would get frustrated when an instance would pop into my mind and evoke the same hard emotions all over again. These were things I thought I had forgiven and moved on from. It felt like all the work I had done to move on was slowly draining down a leaky sink plug. I was angry with myself for not being able to do the work.

It makes sense though, doesn't it? My value came from how hard I could work and what results I could get. I could outperform any day, anywhere, except in my own heart. The more I realized I couldn't body slam my way through the work, the more discouraged I felt. It was only when I surrendered to it all—the emotions, the messiness, the process— that the work didn't seem so overwhelming. When I opened my hands to stop working so hard and allowed myself to be worked on.

When it came to the work, I had been using a high-power pressure washer. When I surrendered, Jesus came in with a broom. I am still new to this approach, but I can say with assurance this type of healing is more profound, impactful, and impressed into my spirit.

If you are body-slamming through your healing, desperately trying to make headway, I want to encourage you to slow down. Sit down. Invite Jesus to sit with you, then open the door to the big and scary emotions on the front porch. It is so beautiful when you let them in and sit with them for a minute. You realize they aren't as bad as you thought they would be. Or maybe your counselor is sitting with you, and you are working through some really big and painful emotions, the type of emotions that make you want to bury your head in the sand. Then, you survive. You are stronger than you realized. Right now, you might want to run, but as long as you keep showing up with open hands, you win.

LEARNING FROM YOUR MISTAKES

Just as there has to be room for healing, patience, and self-compassion on your journey, there also has to be room for mistakes.

From as far back as I can remember, I have beat myself up for my mistakes. One of the ways I used to make money was by cleaning and organizing other people's homes. I had this one cleaning client with so many trinkets and frail décor. When I first started working with her, I was so nervous I kept breaking things, and I became more nervous. It became a vicious cycle, and I ended up breaking something four cleaning sessions in a row! Each time, I would have to face her and tell her what I had broken. It was so embarrassing. For me, one of the hardest things about cleaning was telling a client I had broken something.

The first time I had to tell her, it was hard. It was even worse the second and the third time. I was getting so anxious. I was waiting for her to finally break and get mad at me. I couldn't believe the grace she had every time. She showed me that it was no big deal to her, but I couldn't let myself believe it. I kept putting more and more pressure on myself, and finally, I remember the day, I had to tell her once again what I had broken. Instead of getting mad, she told me she knew the Lord was with me while I was cleaning. She was smiling and hugging me. This was the moment all my fear fell away. That was the last time I ever broke anything. I finally believed my mistakes weren't too big for her.

God used her graciousness to teach me and help me break this pattern of condemning myself. Something switched in me that day. Her grace for me was so consistent I finally trusted it enough to beat my fear.

I have grown so much in my ability to be in relationships without living in fear of consequences and retaliation. I can make a mistake without internalizing it and having it take away from who I am and my core values. My mistakes don't define me.

It has been a long road of unlearning, and I know I'm not at the end. I have hopes for the day I can love myself without judgment, shame, and guilt. I am thankful for how far I have come, and I know God has big things for me. He desires my freedom even more than I do.

One of the main points John Maxwell makes in his book *Sometimes You Win—Sometimes You Learn* is to evaluate your mistakes. He says to not judge yourself for making the mistake but to use the mistake to propel yourself forward.[10] This is the step I most often get hung up on. A lie that

---

[10] Maxwell, *Sometimes You Win—Sometimes You Learn*.

had power in my life for way too long was, "I should have known better." I have to remember to step outside myself—my embarrassment, shame, or guilt—and learn. It can be a lot of work to unlearn these types of lies. Oftentimes, we don't even know why we believe them. That's why it's so important to name the lies and false beliefs, ask for forgiveness, and ask God to show you the truth.

Brené Brown says, "Shame is a focus on self, while guilt is a focus on behavior. This is not just semantics. There's a huge difference between *I screwed up* (guilt) and *I am a screwup* (shame)."[11] I had to learn to separate my worth from my mistakes. This doesn't mean we won't make mistakes. Hopefully, it means we aren't living on the edge, waiting for our next mistake. When we separate our worth from our mistakes, they come and go without knocking us off our feet.

Let your mistakes teach you, not define you.

HAVING IT ALL TOGETHER AS PARENTS AND PEOPLE

A lot of parents want to be their kid's hero, and they think that means they have to have it all together. I am proposing the opposite: our kids can learn more from seeing us make mistakes gracefully. Pretending we "have it together" can be isolating and disconnecting. When we pretend we don't make mistakes, we put distance between us and other people.

An example of this was when my husband, Dakota, told me about a mistake he made while selling our car. He forgot to report the sale on our end, so we got stuck with a parking ticket from the new owner. It was a silly mistake, and he was annoyed at himself about it.

Looking back, I see now that as our daughter watched us have this conversation, she was, likely subconsciously, learning how to handle her mistakes. She was learning how to treat herself when she makes mistakes.

This is why it is so important to be careful with your words. Be careful what you say about yourself because this is how your children or the next

---

[11] Brené Brown, *Rising Strong: How the Ability to Reset Transforms the Way We Live, Love, Parent, and Lead* (New York: Random House, 2015), 194.
Chapter 3

generation are learning to talk about themselves. Your influence can be good or bad, and it's your decision which one it will be.

A sidestep here: We have to use discernment when having honest conversations with our children. Transparency is not an excuse to put our problems or fears on them, even when done unintentionally. Our kids should not be responsible for solving our problems or filling our insecurities. When done in a mindful way, it can be a powerful experience for our children to see us figuring life out, admitting our faults, humbly apologizing, and taking responsibility for our mistakes. Done in the wrong way, it can be more harmful than helpful.

This translates to our everyday life with other people as well. There is a never-ending list of why we feel pressured to "have it all together." We want to be loved, respected, admired, appreciated, accepted, promoted, and the list goes on. When we let down our walls and admit our mistakes, it allows us to have a deeper connection with others. We are showing what it is that makes us human. When we stop trying to be perfect, we realize how much we have in common and can support each other better. For us to be able to take off our mask with other people, we first have to take it off for ourselves.

GIVING YOURSELF CREDIT

We are all on a lifelong journey of healing and growth. Every so often, you should give yourself credit for how far you've come. We don't want to stop focusing on the growth, but stopping once in a while to acknowledge your accomplishments is so refreshing and can give you the motivation to press on.

I have already disclosed that I am type A. I want it all done yesterday. This came up on my husband and I's last vacation. We were taking some time away from our day-to-day lives to talk about the hard stuff: patterns we've had our whole marriage (eight and a half years by that point). It was easy to get discouraged. Why did we still have these same patterns? Why weren't we past this already?

When I looked back at our first and second years of marriage, I remembered that if we had even tried to talk about these same topics back then, they would hurt us so much more and we would both shut down much more quickly. It was all a part of the process. Even if the progress seemed small, we had improved and grown. Looking back and acknowledging our growth gave us the hope we could keep growing and improving.

Give the process credit. It can be hard to be patient and embrace the journey, but it is shaping us.

BREAKING OUT OF COMFORTABLE

Why aren't people creating the life they have always dreamed of? Because somewhere along the way, the work defeated them. They don't know what the work is supposed to feel like. I am here to tell you it is supposed to feel *uncomfortable*. It will be uncomfortable, but it's important to keep pressing on. Keep reading and listening to other people's stories of how they came to success. They will inspire you and confirm you are making progress. You are going in the right direction. You have what it takes. You have the strength.

Have you ever heard the phrase "failing forward"? "Failing" doesn't equal a lack of progress. It's a sneaky tactic of Satan's to convince us that anything that's not a guaranteed success is a waste of energy. We are so easily convinced to stay comfortably where we are rather than be uncomfortable and move forward. With the right mindset, failure can propel you forward. It gives you experience, and if stewarded well, it will make you stronger than before.

Be a victor. Own your choices and your life. Own the journey you are on. Be courageous enough to go head-to-head with failure so you can live the life you've dreamed of.

ACTION:

1. Make a list of qualities or skills you would like to grow in. Take note of the characteristics of the people you admire and ask them how they cultivated that quality.

2. What are three things you feel proud of in your journey?

3. What lies do you believe when you make a mistake? How do you keep your mistakes separate from your worth?

4. What have you pulled back from because it feels like you failed too many times?

HOW DO YOU DEFINE SUCCESS?

Have you ever heard the metaphor about what wall your ladder is on? It's the idea that we're all climbing a ladder, but many people don't take the time to evaluate where they will be when they reach the top. They don't take the time to see if that's actually where they want to be.

A lot of people lean their ladder on the career wall. They climb the ladder for forty years, and in the end, they are frustrated that they aren't where they thought they'd be when they reached the top. They didn't consider the destination before they put in the work.

Instead, let's work backward. Let's begin with the results and work back to what we need to do today, this week, this month, and this year to get those results. I highly recommend the book *The One Thing* by Gary Keller and Jay Papasan to walk you through this thought process.

For many years, I defined success as owning a business. I started my own cleaning and organizing business, worked as an independent contractor, and had a network marketing business. These were the main stamps of approval for me. I felt lost if I couldn't point to measurable accomplishments and prove exactly how much I was worth. It was the pride that came from saying, "Look at what I'm doing. Look at what I've accomplished." This type of thinking is a stumbling block. All that running and striving and working never really gave me worth. Maybe I felt validated while I had a title to point to, but it wasn't true security. That way of living demanded that I stay in motion to keep proving.

This is exactly what the Enemy of our soul wants, for us to stay in motion, lost and chasing lies. Jesus is inviting us to rest, put away the hustle, and just be. He is enough, and I am enough in Him. That is why my year of rest was such an important lesson for me. My hustle was revealing my insecurity. That doesn't mean the people living in the rest and security of Jesus aren't changing the world—they are. There's a difference between hustling and being on a mission. Once you are firmly planted in your value as a child of God, you'll run so fast, but it will be so different. It will be like walking on clouds. Running with passion and purpose within God's will is freeing. It's exhilarating.

When my husband would get home from work each day, I used to list all the things I had accomplished: I did the laundry and the dishes, went grocery shopping, weeded the flower beds, painted the dresser, took the recycling to the center, washed the car, oh, and took care of our three-month-old baby. He'd say he didn't know how I did so much in one day. Now I look back and wonder, "How did I do so much in one day?" Even after doing all that work back then, I would still hit the pillow at the end of the day thinking I didn't do enough. Now it's a good day if we get out of the house before 9:00 a.m. and get three things done. The difference is I feel like I lived more life in one year of rest than I did in the previous five, just by slowing down.

I lived at a pace that was impressive to others but damaging to me. For so long, it was too scary to let go of that lifestyle. I needed other people to believe the good about me so I could believe it about myself. This was not a sustainable way to live. I gave others the power to change how I thought about myself. When you live like this, when people speak highly of you, it boosts your self-worth, but when they don't, any self-esteem you have can be lost in one fell swoop. That begins the cycle all over again. You start running and looking for validation. You start digging in, grinding your teeth, and running harder, faster, and longer to prove you are worth it.

Looking back now, I feel sad for that girl. I'm still not that far removed from her. I want to hug her and tell her: "You are loved. You can stop running. You are safe. You are enough. You have unique gifts and talents the world needs, and you can't fully use those gifts and talents until you stop running. It is okay to declare your worth. It isn't your responsibility to make everyone else comfortable."

If this were a movie, this is the point when the main character would break down and cry because they don't want to keep running, but they don't know how to stop. Getting to that uncomfortable place is the first step.

In my season of rest, I was challenged from so many angles. I was challenged to find my worth in who I am, not in what I do, and to find a definition of success with a foundation in God, not in my to-do list. I am not done yet, but I am so thankful I took the invitation to rest. I feel like Jesus put out His hand and invited me to walk this hard path so I could be whole. I believe deep in my core that God gave me the gift of entrepreneurship and will use it for His glory, but He had to break some old mindsets first.

Don't strive for the world's definition of success; define what success means to you. Evaluate what's important to you, and make sure it's what you truly value, not the world's definition of value that was plopped into your lap and never challenged. It took time and a lot of courage for me to acknowledge my ladder was on the wrong wall. Getting off the wrong ladder isn't easy. You don't want to give up on the work you've put in so far. You worry you're leaving behind all that work for no reason.

If you can jump off that ladder, you'll be free to climb the ladder that will make you happy and fulfilled.

LIVING FOR HERE AND LIVING FOR ETERNITY

Finding what success means to you requires stepping back from the world's definition of success and stepping into what success looks like for a child of God.

This is something that tugs at me. I am a driven person. I enjoy creating systems and making things more effective and efficient. I enjoy the challenges of this life (except when I don't). I struggle with getting too gung ho about my next business or goal. I can get so caught up thinking about my dream house or other materialistic goals. Those things don't matter to our eternal future. I want to make an impact in this world, but I want it to have an eternal impact.

A few years ago, I got a massage from an overseas missionary who does massage as her ministry. She comes back to the U.S. once a year and gives massages to raise funds for their missions overseas. When she is abroad, she runs a massage school and teaches other women this trade. I was honored to get an appointment with her when she was in the U.S.; she has been doing this for ten years and always has a booked schedule when she is in the States.

It was a two-hour massage, and we talked the whole time. At one point, she asked me if I felt called to missions. I said, "No, but I love business. I can make money from anything I look at." Her response was, "Aw, you're a sender." She was referring to Romans 10:15: "And how will anyone go and tell them without being sent? That is why the Scriptures say, 'How beautiful are the feet of messengers who bring good news!'"[12] She was talking about the people who financially support missionaries and help make their work possible. We didn't stay on this subject for too long, but what she said greatly impacted me.

I will admit I haven't always had the right motives for making money. I have often felt guilty about putting my energy and focus into making money, and rightfully so. I wanted it to be for good, but my value was too wrapped up in it. That has been a huge part of my journey, stripping my security and identity from making money.

This is something I am continuously working on, but I've had a change in perspective. God wants me to use my gifts for His glory instead of my pursuit of validation. When I do that, I don't need to feel guilty, embarrassed, ashamed, or worldly because I know my efforts will be used for eternal impact.

Sharing this gift and the money I make with it doesn't always come naturally to me. I have to break out of the scarcity mindset that makes me want to hold on to my resources. When I am able to break through this mindset, I find that I love giving. It fires me up to learn about organizations and nonprofits making an impact. I want to support the organizations acting as the hands and feet of Jesus—they can make an exponential impact if they have the funding. By funding these missions, we allow the staff to keep their heads down and focus on the mission instead of getting distracted by the details. This is so important because when people are living in their strengths, so much more fruit can come from the same amount of effort.

When you are living by the world's definition of success, the goal of

---

[12] Romans 10:15 (New Living Translation).

making money is to be the one with the most at the end of the day. When we are living by God's definition of success, it is about giving that money away and living to the fullest of our potential.

One person working in their strength is more effective than ten people doing the same job out of their strength.

100% AME

There are a variety of studies that show how important visualization is. I like to use this tactic to imagine the most ideal and successful version of myself, the one who is living fully in her purpose. I call her 100% Ame. (Ame is the nickname my cross country team gave me in high school.) When I think of 100% Ame, I see my most beautiful, confident, ambitious, relaxed, graceful, light, and loved version of myself.

I was journaling one day, and this image of 100% Ame just came out. It's how I imagine myself with no negative limitations. This is the entry:

> *When I think of myself as feeling beautiful, I think of my nails done, a messy braid or my warrior princess hair (crimped), my Gap jeans, in bare feet or flat shoes, and a plain T. My bracelets and special necklace, all the stud earrings. And a toe ring. And a belly button piercing. I love piercings. Maybe another tattoo. Just envisioning this makes me feel pretty. I just want to be free. I think it makes me feel free-spirited, sexy, light-hearted, playful, beautiful, spontaneous, fun, laughing, carefree, safe, dancing, playful, present, enjoying life, beautiful, mommy, confident, intelligent but not sternly professional, surprisingly insightful and competent, comfortable with who I am, not making time pass but enjoying the passing time, soaking in the life opposed to making it happen. Cleansed, clean, light, toned, strong, fit.*
>
> *She is in there.*

I did not alter my thought process for you guys.
Sometimes, I can live in this vision of myself without a second thought.

Other times, I have to fight with all my strength to believe the good about myself. I have to fight off the voices that want to take those 100% Ame moments away. I know that eventually, I will be living in that image 24/7. That's what I'm fighting for.

Sharing 100% Ame with you makes me feel vulnerable, but I know there is someone out there who needs to learn to fight for themselves. Don't settle for what other people say you are. Don't let their judgments keep you from living the highest you. Philippians 4:6–8 says:

> Don't worry about anything; instead, pray about everything. Tell God what you need, and thank him for all he has done. Then you will experience God's peace, which exceeds anything we can understand. His peace will guard your hearts and minds as you live in Christ Jesus. And now, dear brothers and sisters, one final thing. Fix your thoughts on what is true, and honorable, and right, and pure, and lovely, and admirable. Think about things that are excellent and worthy of praise.[13]

When I feel stuck, I embrace the image of 100 % Ame and make a decision. I do this when it comes to treating myself. I have a hard time doing even a little something special for myself, whether it is getting a drink from a coffee stand, ordering a side when we are eating out, or grabbing an item off the impulse rack at the grocery store. 100% Ame knows she is worthy of being treated. She is worthy of everything good God has given us in this life.

Harnessing the image of 100% Ame helps me feel worthy, brave, loved, whole, valuable, and authentic.

I hope you are brave enough to imagine this strong version of yourself and embrace it more and more through your journey of growth.

---

[13] Philippians 4:6–8 (New Living Translation).

THE IMPORTANCE OF MINDSET

So many of us define our abilities and limitations by what we own, where we live, and what our economic status is. Really, our mindset is key to whether we are truly successful or not.

You might live in a low-income neighborhood but have a million-dollar mindset. Or you might live in a million-dollar neighborhood but have a low-income mindset. Success can't be achieved just by getting out of a certain neighborhood. You have to get past the mindset of the neighborhood. You can be full of self-worth, purpose, and success despite your circumstances. On the opposite end, you can be living a life of excess but be held back by a mindset of scarcity.

An example of this comes from the movie *The Greatest Showman* and the main character, P.T. Barnum. He grew up as the son of a tailor and living in poverty, and because of this was treated poorly by the man who would one day become his father-in-law. After P.T. Barnum grows up and achieves wealth and success, his father-in-law comes to his now-famous performance. As they talk during the after-party, P.T. Barnum reveals through a stabbing comment that he is still angry and resentful toward his father-in-law after all these years. The father-in-law's response is, "All that fortune and still just the tailor's boy."[14] He is referring to P.T. Barnum's mindset. He is saying that after all he has created for himself, it hasn't changed what he believes about himself.

There is a misconception that if we acquire the dream house, car, and lifestyle, then we won't be so stuck in our old negative patterns. Having "the life" doesn't mean your mindset has changed. It merely means it is hidden. If we're not careful, we'll get caught up in the material things we think will make us happy without growing and evolving on the inside.

While you're building up your life, you also have to be building up yourself and your self-worth. They have to go hand in hand. This is where it comes down to hardcore introspection. You could be fooling everyone around you. You could even be fooling yourself. I was fooling myself for a long time. I was proud of what I had built, but I was missing the component

---

[14] *The Greatest Showman,* directed by Michael Gracey (Twentieth Century Fox, 2017). <u>Chapter 4</u>

of self-esteem. It took me years and some extreme circumstances to be real with myself. I hope you don't have to hit a wall before you see this.

It is often the people who don't think this applies to them that need this balance corrected in their lives most. These things aren't solved in a single day. For now, just leave the door open and acknowledge that something in your life may need to be tweaked. Rest and pray about it first. Praying will open you up to the truth. Ask a few people to tell you what patterns they see in your life. Make sure your heart is open before you approach those people. If you want true feedback, make sure you are willing to receive it. You always have the authority to disagree, but it is your responsibility to do the work.

This book is a tool to help you grow out of your stinkin' thinkin.' You should never deny where you came from, and you should never give excuses for why you're not further in life. Don't make excuses for your lack of progress, but don't judge the speed of your progress. It's about being empowered where you are at.

WHY DON'T WE SHARE
WHAT WE KNOW?

A huge part of success is sharing your skills, wisdom, and purpose with those around you, but I have found time and time again people are hesitant to share what they know. They don't think what they're doing is "cool," has potential for profitability, or would be competitive in the market. They might have a million other reasons that they don't share their gift. Sometimes they see a path that works for someone else, and they are drawn toward that instead. I'll tell you right now, it's a mistake.

God designed you for a specific role. He gave you desires and interests to glorify Him. There's a false belief that our callings from God won't be desirable or fun. Some have been led to believe the lie that the things God will call us to will be hard work and without joy. We think we will have to suffer for our purpose. The reality is the best thing you have to share with the world is the thing you are naturally good at and enjoy.

There was a gal I once knew who dried a certain type of weed that grew on her property and made it into an oil that relieves itches and stings. It was amazing, but she was modest about it. I told her how amazing her oil was, but she told me about another business in town that already sold similar products. I was shocked this was the reason she wasn't selling her product. There is so much room in the world to have success, even if someone else is already doing the same thing.

This woman would admire my skill of cleaning and organizing while underplaying her own talents. She wanted to learn to do what I did. Based on her location alone, it wouldn't have made sense. Even more profoundly though, it wouldn't make sense because she already had an incredible skill to share with the world; she didn't need to do what I did. I so wish everyone had as much admiration for their God-given gifts as they have for other people's gifts. This would be a world of people living in their strengths!

I began my cleaning and organizing business because someone wanted me to clean their house, they named the price, and I agreed. Soon, that person introduced me to some of their connections, and I quickly formed a network of my own.

At first, I didn't have the confidence to advertise that I organized. I didn't see the value in my organizing skills, and I only organized if I was asked. After a while, I started leaning into my specialty of organizing and almost doubled my rate. I was shocked to find the clients I got at my new rate appreciated me even more. When I valued myself, other people valued me too.

I had to fight the urge to pinch myself because I couldn't believe people were paying me to do this. I was working in my strength so much that I was energized by what I was doing. The work felt easy breezy, but I was making money doing it. That is what we all should be experiencing. There are challenges, yes. There will be problems you have to solve, yes. When you are in your strength, it will be hard to believe people are paying you, and you will even be able to charge more than ever.

The wild thing is it might feel weird to charge more because the work comes so naturally to you, but that is why you are worth the extra cost. Would you rather pay more for someone to cut your hair when that skill comes naturally to them, or pay less but be worried the whole time that your hairdresser might cut their fingers? It is human nature to be at ease when someone looks comfortable doing their skill. We are drawn to people who have a humble confidence.

So, share your thing. What comes naturally to you? What activity do you enjoy so much it makes the time fly by? There is likely something you're already doing that would be highly valued by the right audience. You don't have to search wide and far or gain new skills. Your opportunity is right there.

There is this feeling. It has a name: impostor syndrome. I lived there far too long. That's where the Enemy wants you. He doesn't want you to believe your natural gifts and talents have any value. He wants to steer you as far away as possible from the thing right under your nose. He wants you to believe your skills are small and not valued. These are lies.

It is a self-fulfilling cycle. The more you live in your strength and gain confidence in your skill, the more people will support and encourage your talent. The more people that believe in and appreciate what you have to offer, the more confidence you'll have to do the thing, and it just keeps growing.

Don't worry about what other people think. Live in your strength. Shine your light. Live in your purpose. It is magnetic.

ACTION:

1. What wall is your ladder on now? What will the results be when you get to the top? Is that what you want, or do you need to switch walls?

2. Are you living and working in your strengths? Are you using your strengths to make an eternal impact?

3. Visualize 100% you. What does it look like? Jot down the words that come to mind. I encourage you to dig into whatever your chosen form of art is and run with this. Let the creativity inspire you to identify different aspects of 100% you. Not just characteristics, but your whole self.

4. This is the fun part: start dreaming. What are the results you want in life? Now work backward. What would need to happen for that to be possible? Write down your dream.

(4)

GOD HAS SUCH BIG PLANS FOR YOU

For a few years now, I have been letting the motto "Live loved" shape my journey. I feel like it says everything, and I could write a whole book on just those two words.

Honest, passionate, determined, creative, artistic, brave, persistent, intelligent, caring, bold, deep, leader, strong, thoughtful, and teachable.

Living loved means believing all these things for yourself and more.

What we believe about ourselves will determine our choices in life. Our brains are so powerful—it is important to have good thoughts and beliefs about yourself. If I'm being completely honest, it scares me a bit to be writing to future people who will read this and hopefully be empowered to change the way they think about themselves. I want you to not just raise your expectations for yourself, but to truly believe in yourself. The achievements will come when you believe you can accomplish them. You have to believe you are worth what you are achieving. When we overcome our negative beliefs about ourselves, it's like the waters part. I've learned to believe God has such big plans for me. Now I want you to believe God has such big plans for you.

When this new "Live loved" motto was sinking into my heart, I knew it was meaningful to me, but during a conversation with a friend, I realized the seed was even deeper than I knew. Words flowed out of me I didn't even know were in my heart. I came up with so many examples of how I could live differently if I were living loved: If I were living loved, I could be patient and understanding instead of protective or defensive. If I were living loved, I could accept the love and friendship of others instead of sabotaging or deconstructing a positive experience. I could offer positivity, compliments, and praise without needing it to be returned. I could stand firmly in my convictions and not look to others for validation. I could live with a ridiculously loud voice without needing to speak. I could live fearlessly. Living loved is such a quiet strength.

There are so many ways life would be freer if we lived loved. So many people are living out of insecurity and fear, hoping and longing for love to be returned. Our culture has it so backward. I had it backward. Once we start living in the love and acceptance we already have, yes, it will attract people to love us, but we won't be searching for it. Loving authentically is the overflow of living loved.

When I look at my daughter, especially in this season, I think, "God, help me raise a child who knows how loved she is." One of my biggest hopes is that even in my brokenness and lack, she would feel unconditionally loved. I often find myself praying, "God, fill in the gaps where I fall short."

Ultimately it will be His love that fulfills her longing to be loved. I want to give her everything I can while pointing her to the One who will never leave her wanting.

Years ago, I came across a question that stopped me in my tracks: "Are you willing to do less and be more?" Honestly, I still fight against this idea. Some of the lies I have struggled with are that I am unlovable and a burden. The lies we believe in childhood can shape our lives if we don't unlearn them and seek the truth.

Guys, it is hard work to believe the truth, but if we don't fight, we are right where the Enemy of our souls wants us. God isn't asking us to be perfect—He is asking us to keep moving forward. As long as I am willing to lean in, He will use me.

Living loved has opened up a whole new world. Living loved allows me to say no. Living loved allows me to rest. Living loved gives me permission to stop hustling. Living loved allows me to hold my boundaries regardless of how other people act. Living loved has given me strength and courage.

Through this journey, the goal is to shape your mindset and habits around living loved. Keep coming back to this.

FINDING HAPPINESS WHERE YOU'RE AT

I have longed to start a farm for years. My husband and I both thought that when we bought our first house, it would be on a property of at least five acres where we would have room to establish the farm. That did not happen. In 2018, we ended up with just over one-tenth of an acre and very near downtown Spokane, WA.

We bought our house thinking it was just a stepping stone. We were not planning to get established there for two reasons: One, we felt we needed a larger property to realize our dream of the farm. Two, we didn't feel like our neighborhood was ideal. After two and a half years of living in this house, the housing market had risen significantly, and we had landscaped the yard and done some other work on the house. We had a significant amount of equity and thought it was time to move on.

We were one day away from listing our house. We had signed the papers and were ready. I sensed my husband was hesitating. Soon, it became clear to me we weren't moving. I was angry. We split ways from the realtor in October of 2020. Letting go of our plans felt defeating to me. Our dream felt out of reach and indefinitely postponed. I was discouraged, to say the least. I brought my anger to God and began asking Him, "Why are we here?"

I felt stuck, but I also knew I didn't want to live in this negative pattern anymore. I had to make a choice. I didn't want to feel miserable, and since we were now committed to staying here, I chose to change my attitude. I had to choose to be happy. So, I started opening my hands to the plan He had for us here.

God was just getting started.

I had been holding on with closed fists to the idea that we had to move to be happy. I was desperate to have control over my situation. Now that we were staying, happiness was about holding out open hands and receiving what God had for us. I had to let go of control and choose to be okay. Actually, more than okay: peaceful.

With my obsession to have control, I was wringing every last ounce of divinity out of my life. There was no room for God to move because I had to know how things were going to go. God has way bigger plans for us than we could ever have for ourselves. We can only receive them when we let go of having control.

When we first decided to stay in our house, I felt so far away from my dream farm. I had to change my mindset about that too. I hadn't been investing in our property because I was waiting for *the* property. I hadn't been fully committed to living here. I was pushing to get to the next chapter instead of living in this one. Ironically, when I submitted to putting down my plans and timeline for moving, God gave us a farm right here. Now, we have our own urban farm right here in downtown Spokane.

Once I gave up needing to move, I could dream about what we could create here. The creativity started flowing. When I surrendered to being here, to doing the work God has for us here, it was like the floodgates of abundance opened.

A big part of establishing a farm is having the right equipment and tools. I was gifted a number of bee boxes by a beekeeper who was downsizing. I got an excellent deal on all kinds of fencing from someone who was taking down their chicken coop. I got recycled crates to use as raised garden beds.

Then, I saw a brand-new greenhouse on Facebook Marketplace for half the original price. When I saw it, it had already been listed for a day. I told my husband I didn't think there was any way it would still be available, but if I got a phone call, I would buy the greenhouse. The seller called me the next day. She explained she was committed to not just selling the greenhouse but finding it a home where it would be treasured. I was her top pick out of many inquiries. On top of that, she would deliver!

We were gifted chickens and a coop from friends who were moving out of state. We got sheet metal and wood from a barn that was being remodeled. I had been on the lookout for raspberries for a while and was supposed to meet with someone who was selling them for two dollars per cane. For some reason, I stopped hearing from her. I was disappointed. Not even a week later, I found someone giving away a whole patch of raspberries for free.

So many things came together so beautifully; I couldn't have planned it better. Every time another detail came together, I felt more and more that God had given us this farm.

When I get an idea about something, I push hard until I see that thing completed. This journey was different because the farm wasn't something I made happen. Jesus just kept giving and giving, and I couldn't even brag about it in my own power. At the beginning of my season of rest, God gave me the verse Deuteronomy 8:16–18: "He did this to humble you and test you for your own good. He did all this so you would never say to yourself, 'I have achieved this wealth with my own strength and energy.' Remember the LORD your God. He is the one who gives you power to be successful."[15]

I am so thankful we finally chose to embrace the farm here. It has already been so blessed.

BEING THE LIGHT WHERE YOU ARE

When we were in the final week of prep before listing our house, I was so done with our neighborhood. I was done with the size of our house and the lack of land. I was done with the cleaning. I was done with our kitchen seeming so dysfunctional. I was done with everything to do with this house. I had gotten in the mindset that our neighborhood wasn't safe, and I was letting it take over my mind. When we decided to stay, I had to change my mindset.

The biggest thing I had to change was the death I was speaking over our neighborhood. This didn't happen overnight. It began with being mindful of how I spoke. I often found myself saying, "It doesn't feel safe." And guess what? I noticed everything that affirmed that belief. Now, I pray for protection for every square inch of our property and for our cars. I imagine the wall of protection the Lord puts around our property. Things still happen that are less than comforting, but I have worked to change my focus.

Another major thing clicked for me one day. I didn't hear it audibly, but it was so clear God was telling me, "Instead of letting the darkness bring you down, be the light." It made so much sense—how had I not seen it before? These words changed my whole perspective. I began to see my neighborhood as my mission field.

Then I read the book *The Circle Maker* by Mark Batterson. This book references the Bible story of the fall of Jericho, where the people of Israel circled Jericho for seven days until the walls of the city came crashing down. Mark discusses how in this same way we need to circle our dreams with prayer. He invites us to physically walk circles while praying and claim the promises of God.[16]

---

[15] Deuteronomy 8:16–18 (New Living Translation).

[16] Mark Batterson, *The Circle Maker: Praying Circles Around Your Biggest Dreams and Greatest Fears* (Grand Rapids: Zondervan, 2011).

One of the factors getting me so discouraged about this neighborhood was the litter. The prompting from Mark Batterson's book challenged me to claim this neighborhood and to circle it in prayer—while picking up garbage. Now we do "garbage walks," where we walk around the neighborhood and pray while picking up litter. It's a practical way to love our neighbors. On our very first garbage walk, we circled our seventeen-block neighborhood. We prayed and asked that God would open hearts and doors.

About halfway through the walk, a gentleman approached and walked right up to my face. I was a bit taken aback, but I asked, "How can I help you?" He said, "I love what you're doing. You can use my dumpster anytime. I own the recycling center."

Wow. What an incredible answer to our prayers and confirmation we were on the right path. I felt God so clearly telling me, "I didn't put you here to get you down. I put you here to fight for this neighborhood."

When we were buying this house, the sellers decided to sell it to us for much less than they could have on the market. We questioned them, asking them if they really wanted to do this. They responded, "It's a God thing. We believe this house is yours."

From the very beginning, it was always God's plan for us to live here. We claimed that. We knew God gave us this house. Just because the journey is hard and bumpy doesn't mean it isn't God's plan. It took me almost three years to submit to the reasons God placed us here. I selfishly thought He gave us this house so we could have the equity to move on to a new house sooner. This route was the harder one to accept. I've had to come to a place of praising Him for the challenging route. This is the route that made me draw close to Him.

Changing my mindset has been a journey, and I am still in progress. We had an instance right outside our fence that left me feeling out of control and unsafe for about two weeks. It triggered all sorts of insecurities and emotions for me. I desperately wanted the situation to be taken care of, and part of me thought if I was ruthless and harsh, it would get taken care of sooner. Despite my big feelings, the Holy Spirit softened my heart and gave me compassion for the people involved. I was still actively pursuing getting the situation resolved, but I believe my kindness made a lasting impact. I remember the night I broke down on my knees, interceding for this person. I felt such a flood of overwhelming emotion and weight.

This was another breakthrough moment. What if God had us stay just for one person? What if He had us stay to change one person's darkness to light and to point to Him?

You know the prayer, "Break my heart with what breaks yours"? It was like I could feel the heavenly heartbreak. It changed me. To pray for someone I didn't even know with that weight on my heart was radical. I thought if God had kept us here for just one life, it had all been worth it. I don't think that is the case, but I do think God used that experience to open my eyes. God didn't bring us here to crush me in the oppression. He brought us here strategically to be a light.

The longer we lived in this house, the more I began to uncover the beliefs that were causing tension in me. I had so many expectations for myself about the kind of neighborhood I would raise kids in. I was living with so much subconscious disappointment in myself. I didn't even recognize this was a factor in my dissatisfaction until I started doing the deep digging. Looking back, I see how much I was judging myself, thinking I should be further in life and giving my daughter better or more. When I find thoughts like that in my head now, I remind myself this is our mission field. This is where we've been called to be for this season, and our job is to love our neighbors the best we can.

ACCEPTING THE CHALLENGE TO STAY

Choosing to stay in our house was so much more about my attitude than any practical factors. God showed me very clearly if He had given me the dream farm while I was in this state of discontent, I would have been unhappy with it in three years.

We could have moved; we could have made the move happen, but I know deep down if we had done this, I would have skipped an important step. God still had work He wanted to do in me here first. It wasn't like I heard God say, "No, don't move," but I see so clearly now that by trying to move, I was running. I wasn't packed and ready to go because I was seeking God's will. I was done, and I wanted out of the discomfort. I wanted to escape the pain and frustration I was in.

When I finally stopped running and submitted, I saw just how tightly my hands were closed. It still puts me in awe to think about how I had to get to that place of *so done* for God to reveal what He had for me. I had to go through the tension of being ready to leave to learn the lessons of staying. It is easy when it's comfortable. If we had moved, I would have just been pushing off the work that still needed to be done—but God always has an open invitation for us to follow Him and submit.

ALLOW GOD TO DO THE HEALING

In *The Circle Maker*, Mark Batterson says over and over, "Pray like it depends on God and work like it depends on you."[17] I love this because it keeps us with a posture of open hands while still putting weight on our part. I can be on both ends of the pendulum swing, either taking too much credit when I should be giving glory back to God, or on the other end being so "humble" that I put myself down. I love this definition of humility from Ken Blanchard in *Sometimes You Win—Sometimes You Learn* by John Maxwell, "Humility does not mean you think less of yourself. It means you think of yourself less."[18] Be careful you aren't claiming humility while beating yourself up.

God is doing great work in all of us. He never ceases to pursue us. He is constantly inviting us into healing, and we just need to take His lead. We all have a responsibility to take the invitation. Give glory to God, yes, but you also have to take the invitation. God isn't going to force you. He will invite you.

I have fallen so many times in the past, and that is precisely why I'm here. It is why I'm at this place in my journey and why I'm here writing. This twists my mind too much, so I try not to think too hard about it, but when I look back I can see how God has been inviting me on this journey for years. *Years.* I get caught up in wondering how my life would be different if I had said yes sooner. How much pain could I have saved if I just trusted and followed His leading?

Despite all this, I also trust there is a perfect plan, and I am in it. So, trust God, give Him glory, and do the work!

---

17 Batterson, *The Circle Maker*.
18 Maxwell, *Sometimes You Win—Sometimes You Learn*, 25.

ACTION:

1. What would it look like if you lived totally loved? Create a scene. Who would you be if you immersed yourself in living loved?

2. Write at least ten positive characteristics you have. John Maxwell says, "Don't stop until you have written a hundred positive things about yourself."[19] Read them out loud at least once a day.

3. What do you need to open your hands to?

4. Do you have a hope or dream you are *making* happen? What is the next step you could take toward that dream?

____

[19] John C. Maxwell, *The 15 Invaluable Laws of Growth: Live Them and Reach Your Potential* (New York: Center Street, 2012), 49.

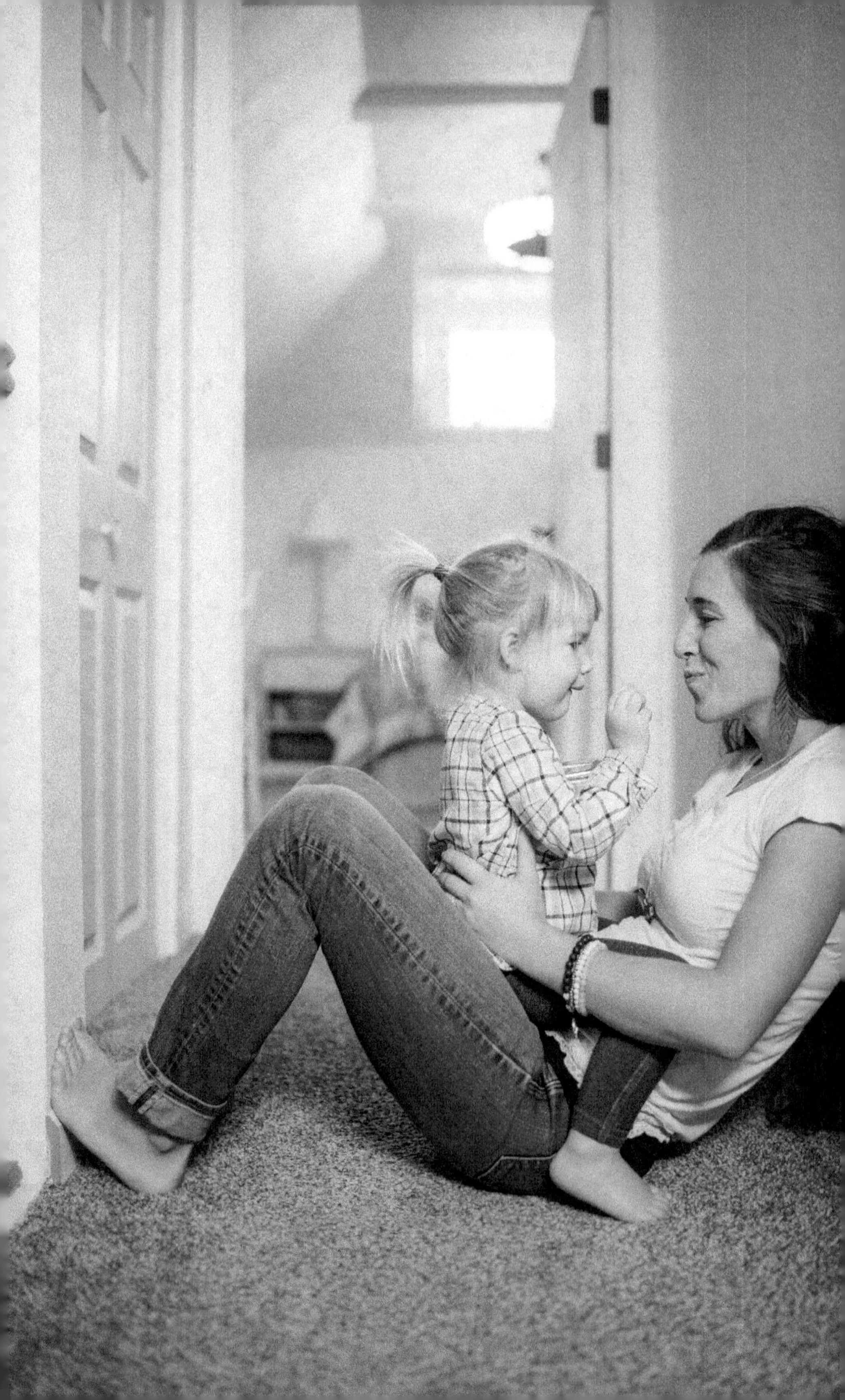

PART 2

RELATIONSHIPS AND COMMUNICATION

5

BUILDING HEALTHY RELATIONSHIPS

I had a running coach in college for one season. When I started working with him, I hadn't competed in two years. He didn't think I should be training with the top three women on the team because he didn't think there was any way I would be able to compete with them after such a big gap in my training. In the first race of the season, I tied with the third-fastest runner. He was shocked by my performance. After that race, he adjusted my workouts and expected way more out of me.

This is another example of how in the past, I have found my strength in proving people wrong, and I want to explore this relationship dynamic more. I thrived off people being surprised that I beat their expectations. Instead of voicing my confidence and calling them out for their low expectations, I waited for the opportunity to prove them wrong. I believed that if I was accepted upfront, I wasn't being authentically accepted. It only felt real if I had to prove myself.

That was my insecurity, and it led to a lot of relationships where I wasn't valued for who I was but what I could offer. I dismissed the people who would accept me as I was and was drawn to those I had to prove myself to. In this way, I was inviting in and reinforcing the pain.

I have had so many conversations with people wondering why they keep attracting the same kind of people into their lives, even though it is precisely the type of person they don't want to form relationships with. This has to do with who we are. We have to dig deep and identify the insecurities we are trying to fill with our relationships, often subconsciously.

These new relationships seem great while both people are being fulfilled. Then something clicks; one event can change the trajectory of the whole relationship. Sometimes, there have been warning flags for a while, but they were ignored because the positive outweighed the negative. This is when, if we aren't careful, a relationship can get toxic.

The way I see it, there are three different types of relationships. There is the first type, in which both people are unaware of the effects of their actions. They are acting and reacting with little to no insight or reflection. They don't know why they're doing what they're doing. They don't know what their negative patterns are or how to make them stop. These relationships are toxic and have the potential to become abusive.

In the second type of relationship, one person is able to see the negative patterns, but when they point those patterns out to the other person, that person chooses to deflect and avoid responsibility. There is an opportunity for both parties to engage, see their insecurities, take responsibility for their actions, and mend the relationship. If only one party is willing to be vulnerable, they set themselves up as a target.

This doesn't always mean that the person not willing to be vulnerable is doing this vindictively. Often it is just immaturity and pride that prevents them from taking down their defenses, and they end up hurting the other person without meaning to. I often see this in partnerships. There are two people who love each other deeply, and one person longs to have a more intimate, emotional connection. They allow themselves to be vulnerable for the success of the relationship, but over time they actually feel more distant from their partner. Every time they choose the path of vulnerability, they are met with harshness, aggression, or defensiveness. (This is the other person's immaturity and pride.) Instead of being vulnerable, they are tightly guarding the gate. I want to believe that most of the time this is done innocently, but that doesn't prevent their actions from being destructive.

There is another danger to this type of relationship: there are people who will take advantage of, manipulate, and exploit a person willing to be vulnerable. They will collect all the information they can by sympathizing with the vulnerable person and then use their wounds as ammunition.

They will gaslight and manipulate further. They aren't matching the vulnerability. They are pulling it out of the victim to use for their benefit.

Be discerning. If you see this pattern start to emerge, don't continue to be vulnerable with that person.

The third and most desirable type of relationship is two people who are willing to look introspectively when conflict arises. You want to be around people who are willing to search within themselves and receive insight and feedback from others. When one person is willing to look at themselves, it helps open the door for the other person to look at themselves too. I know it seems backward, but when the other person sees you are willing to take responsibility for your part, they will feel safe to be vulnerable and look inside themselves.

It can be scary to be the first one to take responsibility. It is a risk because the other person could see your vulnerability as an invitation to walk through the open door and drop their emotional baggage in front of you. I can see them dusting their hands off and thankful you made it so easy for them.

Although there is a potential risk, there is a potential reward as well. By taking responsibility, you could also be setting the stage for a deeper connection. When you are in the right relationship, the other person will meet you halfway. They will open their heart too.

If I am in the third type of relationship, I have a tool I use if an argument gets heated. I ask if I can be vulnerable with them. This question protects both people. It protects me from setting myself up as a target, and it protects the person I love from carrying too much emotional weight when they aren't ready. Sometimes asking the question changes the mood of the argument, and the other person can willingly answer yes, and our connection grows deeper. Sometimes the answer is no because they are not in a good space to hold my heart gently. That is a valid answer, and we can come back to the conversation when things have calmed down, but this method protects both of us.

We often get into unhealthy relationships when we are trying to fill an insecurity in our lives. So how do we stop the cycle? By naming your insecurities and surrendering them to God. Work on building strength and confidence in those areas. Once you can name the insecurity, it's only a matter of time before the battle is won! It will still be hard work, but you have a favorable position.

I have a theory that if you *need* something, you have handed over your power to that thing. I don't want to submit my power to the first person who says I'm pretty, praises my work, laughs at my jokes, thinks I'm wise, etc. I don't want to need anyone's approval, praise, or affirmation.

What is the insecurity you are trying to fill? It's natural to be drawn to people who make us forget that insecurity, even just for a moment. In turn, you might be filling an insecurity for that other person. When those things are revealed, and we recognize we are in the negative pattern again, we have a choice. We can choose to stop living an artificial life, taking the consolation prize for work we didn't achieve, or we can do the hard work of finding authentic relationships.

In our lives, we will have relationships that drain our energy, and we will have relationships that fill us with joy. Seek the relationships that fill you with joy.

You can do this! It will be worth the work. The people you spend time with will change the trajectory of your life. Choose those people carefully.

HOW YOU HELP MATTERS

I don't know about you, but when someone I care about does or says something I view as incorrect, I have the tendency to try and fix the situation for them. Sometimes I can catch myself trying to take the blame and uncomfortable feelings away to make others feel better. This doesn't truly help the other person. Furthermore, it can be damaging to them and to ourselves.

I've had to learn to let the other person sit with their own discomfort and ugly feelings. Before, my programmed response was to take the fault for them. I'd apologize and make whatever it was easier for the other person to fix the discomfort.

As a child, I was stripped of emotional boundaries. I was programmed to admit fault even when I hadn't done anything wrong. I submitted quickly to other people's truth to preserve my safety. I wasn't allowed to think for myself or share my views. I wasn't even allowed to disagree or defend myself. This is not uncommon. I'm here to challenge you to break out of that place. Be bold and brave. Do the work it takes to break those patterns.

There is power in letting someone sit with their mistakes. It's not your responsibility to take on the pain for them, make them comfortable, or even engage in that conversation with them. That is just enabling them, and by doing that, you are giving them the power they're looking for. People who haven't learned to face the consequences of their actions and keep getting a get-out-of-jail-free card have no motivation to change. We are doing a disservice when we take away natural consequences. In their book *Boundaries with Kids*, Dr. Henry Cloud and Dr. John Townsend quote this saying in the context of raising kids, "Nothing happens until the pain of remaining the same is greater than the pain of changing."[20] The way you help matters.

This can happen even in conversation. We don't even have to take physical action to take a person's problem from them. I can only tell you this because I've learned it firsthand. It is hard to let someone— especially the people closest to us—sit in their struggle. I am the person who tries to solve a problem right then during the conversation. I will find all the solutions and do all the work for someone else just to get to the end of the conversation feeling frustrated. As I'm sitting there, wondering why I'm so frustrated, I realize they didn't want a solution. I was doing work that wasn't valued. Some people want to stay stuck in their problems. I have to set down my desire to control the situation. I have to identify what is in my court and what is in theirs.

WHAT'S IN YOUR COURT?

I have used this mental image of a basketball court for years. Imagine multiple basketball courts side by side. You are standing on your court, and the lines are clear. Each person is on their own court. No one can cross your boundaries without consent. You are only responsible for what

---

[20] <u>Chapter 5</u>
Dr. Henry Cloud and Dr. John Townsend, *Boundaries with Kids: When to Say Yes, When to Say No, to Help Your Children Gain Control of Their Lives* (Grand Rapids: Zondervan, 1998), 186.

happens in your court, not for what happens in anyone else's court. No one else is responsible for what happens in your court.

You are responsible for yourself and for your responses and reactions. You are responsible for your emotions, what you eat, how often you exercise, if you get enough sleep, if you get to work on time, etc. You are responsible for your boundaries. You are responsible for who you're going to be, no matter what situation you're in.

I like the basketball court visual for many reasons. One reason is it creates an emotional border that provides safety. I can protect myself no matter how someone else chooses to conduct themselves. I can maintain authority over my choices no matter what they choose. I have power and responsibility over my borders.

I often find myself having to go back to square one and remind myself of what is in my court. Is what I am investing emotional, physical, or mental energy on even my responsibility in the first place? I can evaluate the situation and see if there is any part that is my responsibility or if I would be taking over someone else's problem. I have found so many times that when I'm worked up about something, it's because I'm trying to control something that's not in my court. Once I make that realization, I can let go, take a deep breath, and refocus on what is in my court.

Sometimes there are shared responsibilities, but I get to decide who I share those responsibilities with. Sharing responsibilities is a way to invest in those relationships. Once my part is done and I hand the responsibility over to their court, I don't get to say what they will do with it. I have chosen to give the responsibility willingly, not based on what they will do with it, but my decision to give. That's why it's important to choose these people carefully.

It takes a lot of self-control to not officiate someone else's court. It is easy to get caught up and blur the lines if we aren't being mindful and assertive about what's ours to take responsibility for and what is not. A lot of people will use shame, guilt, and manipulation to try and make something seem like your responsibility. Don't take the bait. Be strong and stand firm in not taking responsibility for what is theirs, especially when they are trying to hand it to you. If you refuse to carry another person's garbage, they may not want to be in a relationship with you. Potentially, and until they become aware of their patterns, they are subconsciously looking for people who will take on their burdens. When you can confidently separate your responsibilities from theirs, you will find the strength to not cave into carrying what isn't in your court.

The visual of the court gives me an emotional border. I can visualize the other person isolated in their court. Whatever emotions are boiling out of them are stuck in their space. My safety, security, and worth are not dependent on what is going on in their court. I do not have to calm or control what is going on in their court to be safe. I can determine how much I let them influence me, and I can choose to disengage. I have found so much strength in my authority to define my boundaries.

When my baby was born, I was in an emotionally vulnerable place. My husband and I decided we were going to enjoy our baby and have no visitors for three days once she arrived. People were anxious to meet her, but I am so thankful we kept this sacred time.

During this time, I had a lightbulb moment. There had been people in my life who I didn't have a healthy relationship with, but I didn't feel like I could enforce boundaries with them. I realized that I needed to protect my baby from these negative patterns, and if I was going to do that for her, why would I not do that for myself?

I had been trying to be a good friend, but all I was being was a garbage dump. This was clear when I pointed out the negative patterns I saw in these relationships. I was willing to work on the relationships but instead was met with the end of these friendships. When I made boundaries, I was no longer wanted. Losing the "friendships" felt so scary to me, which was why I didn't address these issues sooner. I was holding onto something that was hurting me so I didn't make a mess. It's like I was holding onto a pot of oatmeal, and the heat was searing through the oven mitts. The longer you hold on, the worse the burn will be, but letting go will spill oatmeal everywhere. Don't be afraid to spill the oatmeal.

I have chosen to drastically change the emotional weight I let others put on me. I am still empathic, which means I have to be even more aware of and firm with my boundaries. I know I am sensitive to emotional energy. It is a beautiful part of me, and it can be exhausting. I have to steward this part of myself well because I will shut down or break down if I am not intentional about where I'm using my emotional energy. I have to keep evaluating what is in my court and what is in theirs. As I continue to grow in this area, I am getting better at recognizing when I am working outside of my court. Just like everything else, the more you see it, the more you will see it, and then you will see it sooner and sooner.

Imagine if we lived in a world where everyone had to sort their own garbage instead of passing it off to the next person. When we refuse to receive the trash someone is trying to pawn off on us, it takes their power away and can defuse the situation. When we keep our boundaries, it can feel like we are escalating the situation. That's because the other person will become frantic for us to take ownership of their discomfort. Staying in our court gives us the ability to love them better. Brené Brown says in *Rising Strong*, "Compassionate people ask for what they need. They say no when they need to, and when they say yes, they mean it. They're compassionate because their boundaries keep them out of resentment."[21]

PROCESSING INSTEAD OF PASSING

I have a vivid memory of a time I went grocery shopping. I made eye contact with a coach-looking gentleman, and we politely smiled at each other. At that moment, his son came up and tried to help him carry one of the four gallons of milk he had in his hands, accidentally causing his dad to drop one. The dad immediately snapped at the kid. I felt so sad for the kid and the dad. I wanted to hug the child and the child within the father.

The father's reaction was revealing. Our reactions are communicating our wounds. In people's reactivity, they show a piece of their story. They reveal their embarrassment, discomfort, humiliation, etc.

What is your go-to emotion? It is so important that we can label our feelings so we can process them. If we don't intentionally process them, we end up passing them on. If we name them and own them, we can process and apologize instead of blaming and projecting.

I wish it was possible to live 100% loved all the time. Then we wouldn't have to worry about passing on our garbage. I feel especially passionate about parenting out of "living loved." We need to recognize and apologize when we react in a negative way. Our children need to know it isn't their fault when we react out of our own hurt and insecurity.

---

[21] Brown, *Rising Strong*, 115.

You don't have to be perfect. Just keep doing the work of processing and making repairs.

As I'm writing this, my daughter is currently three and a half, and she is amazing. Whenever I catch myself being less than 100% loving to her, I make a point to apologize and tell her how much I love her. I tell her there is nothing she can do to make me love her less. I say in a funny voice, "Babe, I'm losing my patience." She then grabs the air and throws it to me, saying, "I got you more patience." And it works! We end up cracking up. This is a practice we have grown into doing often for each other. It is a great exercise in naming our emotions and having power over them. She throws away the mad or frustration and gets some happiness or obedience instead.

PARENTING EMPOWERED

We had a playdate with a friend and her two girls not too long ago. The girls love being together, and they have so much energy we just let them wear themselves out. This mama has told me about how her girls don't pick up their toys. So when it came time to pick up the mess from the playdate, it was no surprise there was a meltdown.

After the playdate, I went to send a message to this mama to tell her thanks for playing and what a good mama I thought she was. When I got to my phone, I already had a message from her. She was apologetic and embarrassed about her children's meltdown. I could see and feel she was feeling pressure. She was getting sucked into this all-consuming mindset of, "What are people going to think about how I am handling my children right now?" My gut response was to tell her not to feel those things. I wasn't putting those things on you, so let those feelings go. It's okay to evaluate the situation and reflect on what could have gone differently, but don't pick up those negative thoughts.

I don't think anyone can get through parenting without getting sucked into that black hole. Usually, it is a specific atmosphere that will trigger it. For some, it might be within a small group or with the people we perceive as having it together. For some, it might be with our family or people we want to impress. The options are endless. When a situation is overly stressful or stimulating for us as a parent, we need to remind ourselves that we are people too, and we are working through our triggers too.

Living loved means you are the captain of your ship. We tend to look around for approval when we're not confident in our decisions. The way to stay out of the black hole is by educating yourself. Find resources, books, podcasts, and mentors. Know why you are doing what you are doing, and when you don't know, evaluate, process, and make a plan. When you believe and are confident in your decisions, it takes away so many frantic feelings. When you have a plan and know why you are doing it, the plan won't change every five minutes.

There was a season when I found myself so frustrated and lost in parenting. It took breaking down into tears for me to evaluate why. I found I had all the resources I needed. I just needed to be more intentional about using them. We need to commit to action steps.

LOST TIME TO LOVE

As I write this, my husband and I have been married going on nine years. My marriage has been a journey to get to where we are today, and we have come a long way.

We met in seventh grade. He sat in front of me in calligraphy class. He was the new kid, and I was the rebel. We went to the same youth group and got more familiar with each other, but still didn't really know each other. Freshman year, he asked me out twice, and both times I said I just wanted to be friends. I said, "I don't really know you." He was the only boy who was brave enough to be my friend after I turned him down. *Twice.*

He did pursue a friendship with me. I ran cross country, so he did too. We put in a lot of miles and hours together over the next four years. Since time was my love language and running was my favorite hobby, it didn't take long for him to win me over. Sophomore year, he kissed me instead of asking me to date him, and here we are now eleven years later.

There was plenty of drama between the first kiss and "I do," but between the "I do" and our eight-year anniversary, we have struggled through a lot.

We have swung back and forth between madly in love and *How did I fall in love?* so many times. I would get so frustrated because I felt like he wasn't being the man I expected him to be. I felt he wasn't growing, achieving, pursuing something grander, being the spiritual leader, being my partner in business, etc. I would get so frustrated it would make me want to run, hide, shut down, or leave. And that is what I did. It felt safer to run, escape, or leave than to be angry. I wanted so desperately for him to chase me, to pursue me, to see beyond my words, and to fight for me.

Over time, I made choices that put me in a compromising situation. I didn't cross a physical line, but my heart slipped. I was making the type of emotional connection with another man that I should only have with my husband. This broke him, and at the time, I didn't really care. I was so wounded I wanted him to suffer. This is not something I'm proud to share. It hurts me to remember the immaturity and insecurity that made me consider putting aside my marriage and my vows. Unfortunately, it is part of our story, and I hope there is someone out there who can benefit from hearing it.

For so long, I was trying to change my husband. I pushed him away by trying to make him a man I thought I could love more. There should be some accountability for your spouse to learn how to meet your needs, but I found what our relationship really needed was for me to focus on who *I* was being. Once I turned the focus inward and started giving him some credit and praise for what he was doing, it was like he was a whole new man. Sometimes we just need to change the color of our glasses, even if nothing actually changes.

In Stormie Omartian's book *The Power of a Praying Wife*, the first prayer says, "I realize that in some ways he may never change, but at the same time, I release him to change in ways I never thought he could."[22] This is so powerful. I had such strict ideas about what quality my husband needed to change next and the timeline he should do it in, even if only under layers of my subconscious. As I have gotten more flexible with my own healing, allowing God to do things in His own timing, I have gained so much perspective and grace for my husband to be on his own journey. I have found more grace for loving him through his journey.

Without fail, if I try to control the pace of his progress, I end up slowing it down. I end up pushing my husband away and being more frustrated myself. If I backtrack my thoughts when I get in this state, I can see I am acting out of insecurity. My insecurity can quickly shift the focus

---

[22] Stormie Omartian, *The Power of a Praying Wife* (Eugene: Harvest House Publishers, 1997), 42.

from what I need to do to what he needs to do. Let's be real, it's vulnerable to dig into those insecurities. If we don't, then it is just shifting the blame. It is sidestepping responsibility. I can't ask him to put in the effort if I'm not willing to match it. If I lower the standard for me, I lower the standard for us. I want so much more for our relationship. By shifting the blame, I miss out on my own progress.

This is hard for me to admit because sometimes I just want a break from working on myself. Sometimes, I want to be okay with being the immature one.

Dr. Emerson Eggerichs and Sarah Eggerichs say in their *Love & Respect* workbook, "The one who sees himself or herself as the most mature moves first."[23] I don't want to settle for immaturity. I want to be brave, fierce, vulnerable, and authentic. I want to invite my husband into the work and not sit back and hope for someday. I would rather invite him into that and be hurt than give up.

When the progress isn't tangible, it can be hard to maintain self-control. I have to open my hands to the One who is in control and trust that He is working. In the meantime, I can fight for my husband. When I recognize my insecurity, instead of spiraling, I can pray. I have to focus on *what I can do* to keep myself out of the trap I have fallen into so many times.

The good news is that the more you recognize it, the easier it is to switch directions. Author Portia Nelson has a poem called "Autobiography in Five Short Chapters." It is a beautifully simplistic story about a person who walks down a street and falls into a hole. Each time they go on a walk, they get a little bit wiser. First, they recognize they are in a hole and find their way out sooner. Eventually, they avoid the hole. Finally, they choose a different street to walk on.[24]

It took me opening my hands and having patience for my own healing to be able to do the same for my husband. I had to face what wasn't working for me, and that made it so much clearer what wasn't working

---

[23] Dr. Emerson and Sarah Eggerichs, *Love and Respect Conference and 10-Week Study Workbook* (Love and Respect Ministries, 2016), 23.

[24] Portia Nelson, "Autobiography in Five Short Chapters," in *There's a Hole in My Sidewalk: The Romance of Self-Discovery* (Atria Books/Beyond Words). Chapter 6

in our relationship. At the time, I don't even know if I recognized I had a strict agenda for his progress. Now I see my anger was coming from a place of feeling out of control.

Just tonight we were snuggling, and I was brought to tears thinking about all the time I have lost being mad, thinking he wasn't the man I wanted him to be. He is an amazing man. He is on his own journey, and if I would just let that journey unfold, I could be his partner in it instead of a brick in the road he has to keep moving. He is always there for me when I come back and accept him for who he is. He hasn't hardened his heart to me despite all the times I have turned away, waiting for him to be "better." I am so thankful for his compassion and forgiveness.

ACTION:

1. Take five of your closest relationships and identify if they are type one, two, or three relationships. Can you identify any toxic patterns in these relationships?

2. Do you have any relationships where you need to enforce emotional boundaries?

3. Identify a go-to emotion you experience when you are in a stressful situation. Is this an emotion you need to process so you don't pass it on?

4. Can you identify any relationships where you are shifting the blame? Where do you need to take the responsibility to heal and improve your relationships?

6

BE BRAVE ENOUGH TO SAY NO

Many of us are so afraid to ask for help or for the things we want in life that we never ask the questions at all. What are we so afraid of? My theory in life is the worst that can happen when we ask a question is the answer is no.

Reminding myself the worst thing that can happen is the answer is no makes my questions so much easier to ask. I often even say this out loud to the person I'm asking. It's such a great icebreaker!

I love it when I make new friends, meet new neighbors, get business opportunities, have a wish granted, have a mistake undone, get money reimbursed, get a discount, or more just because I asked. Many of these opportunities wouldn't have been possible if I hadn't asked the question in the first place.

Did you know you don't have to let things be awkward? I used to be the queen of being awkward. I didn't have the confidence to assert myself, and I didn't know how to respond when something didn't go the way I'd hoped. I was so timid, I just hoped someone would answer the question I didn't have the courage to ask. It made for a lot of awkwardness.

Luckily, I had role models along the way that gave me tools for communication. One of the best role models I had in my younger years was my cross country coach from high school. She took the scary out of communication and conflict. People bent over backward to get her what she wanted because she was always so nice. She made sure everyone on the team had a vote. She helped the underdog have a voice. She made the options clear and concise. She would agree to disagree instead of invalidating you. She was the master at pros and cons lists. She made the team a safe place for us to say what we needed to say, whether it was to her or to our teammates. She could spot rifts in relationships a mile away, and she refused to let them fester. She not only modeled clear communication, but she walked side by side with us through the hard and messy teenage years, working on it with us.

Something I have learned to take away the awkward is to acknowledge that no is an option right up front. It is funny how reminding people of this seems to kindle a more willing yes. Whenever I return something, I'll walk up to the clerk and say something like, "My theory in life is that the worst that can happen is the answer be no, so I thought I would ask. If it doesn't work out, it's not a big deal, but I was wondering if there is any way I could return this even though I don't have the receipt?" I've already given them the option to say no, so I've lowered the stakes.

I love the way this has changed my approach to life. "No" is more than just a word: it's a mindset. As far back as I can remember, I have had the entrepreneur spirit in me. As a child, I fearlessly asked my neighbors for work. I even sold bracelets at a children's clothing exchange store when I was six. I asked, and they said yes. Over time, that light was put out. I carried a lot of baggage and worries about the retaliation of asking anything. This came from the inconsistency and indirectness with which my questions were answered in the formative years of my life. I closed myself off. By asking questions, I was inviting mistreatment, embarrassment, or misunderstanding. At home and at school, I lost the desire to ask. I didn't know how to handle the frustration, so I put up walls.

High school changed the trajectory of my life. I got to a point where I believed I didn't need anyone else. I began to use my voice, and I began to stand and fight for what I needed. I got to the place where I was owning my future. I don't say this pridefully because now I know that strength came from deep pain. I am so thankful I rose and so sad I thought I had to do it alone.

Even though at the time I felt like I was fighting alone, I see now how surrounded I was by people who were fighting for me, people like my high school coach who served as powerful role models in my life. I am so thankful for the people who fought for me. If you are in a position of influence and you are wondering if what you're doing is making a difference, I'm here to tell you that it is. It was the people who didn't give up on me that impacted me the most. I had teachers, youth leaders, a student advisor, a principal, coaches, and mentors who believed in me beyond what I could believe for myself.

It was a journey to find my voice, regain that confidence, and reshape my mindset. There is so much power and freedom in being able to ask questions boldly.

NO IS A VALID ANSWER

Voicing that no is a valid answer helps me communicate more directly with people. It also helps people communicate more directly with me. It helps people say their real answers. Giving them the option to say no, even though they always had it, helps them realize they can use that option. I have found ways to gently insert the other person's "out." I want people to be direct, clear, and honest. I don't want them to overcommit themselves just to make me happy. I would rather have a no upfront than a strained yes. I would rather have a no now than a yes that is canceled later. I have often found that making no an easy answer helps me feel more confident about their yes.

When I am communicating with anyone, but especially people who may have a hard time saying no, I let them know I will have other options if they say no. I am taking responsibility for my own situation while inviting them to help. For example, I might say, "Hey, I have a dresser in the car I need help carrying inside. Would you be willing to help me with that when you come over on Thursday? If not, it's not a big deal. I have a few other people I can ask, but since I have you, I thought it would be worth asking."

I try to make it as easy as possible for the other person to reject the invitation. I don't want someone to agree to help and wish they hadn't or have a bad attitude about what I've asked them to do.

There are so many times when adults take away the option for a child to say no. I once heard the idea that sharing is something we only ask kids to do. Their theory was that we need to change the verbiage to "taking turns." In an office, you wouldn't complain to your boss that your coworker wasn't sharing their stapler. In all my child-raising experiences, I have enforced that no is a valid option.

I tell my daughter if she wants something, she can ask, but they can say no. When someone asks her for something or if another child takes something from her, I remind her that no is a valid option. There have been many times when I've advocated for the other child. Other parents hearing no is a valid option can help them be gentler with their child too.

Some parents will insist that kids need to share the swing, for example. Yes, taking turns would be kind, but I think it's damaging to teach our children to give up whatever they have any time another person waltzes by and wants what they have.

By voicing to others that no is an acceptable answer, you take down an invisible wall. You make it acceptable for people to say no and evoke a stronger yes.

WITHDRAWING THE INVITATION

When someone is saying yes but their actions are saying no, sometimes I will withdraw my invitation. That is within my court. You don't have to spend time with someone who is saying yes while their body language or attitude is saying no.

By doing this, you are setting the standard for how you want to be treated. A lot of people can feel stuck in this type of situation. Maybe the other person happily agreed two days ago, but now that the day has arrived, they are in a bad mood. I have been in a position so many times where I no longer want the help or company I originally asked for. I didn't believe I had the authority to withdraw the invitation. Now I know I do.

I choose how I will be treated.

Some may argue we need to be there for others on their bad days and love them through it. I agree. My question is, at what expense? We still need to set the standard for how we will be treated. When you are in this type of situation consistently, it is hard to discern when it's a day you need to be there and when it's a day you need to set a boundary. It is when you are in a healthy relationship that you can take time to be an encourager. Unbalanced emotions should be the exception, not the rule.

I noticed a pattern in my life: When I wasn't doing well, I would push everyone away. I'd start making habits and routines to help me get to a better place. After I was doing well again, I would immediately allow negative patterns and people back into my life. I'd let the good habits slip because I was doing well. I would be feeling good and think I could handle it. It would be such a slow backslide that I wouldn't even notice the decline. I would end up depressed and isolated—again.

It was such a big breakthrough when I caught on to this cycle. Setting boundaries doesn't mean you are letting your friends down. We all need cheerleaders sometimes, but sometimes people just want to play the victim instead of doing the work to get back up. I will fight with you, I will contend for you, but I don't want to go down with you. I had to put up boundaries. One of those boundaries is withdrawing invitations.

I want to empower you to use the voice you didn't know you had. You can do this. The more you pick healthy friends and the more you see the negative patterns, the less you will have to use this tool.

An image comes to mind of a floaty with bricks on top of it. A floaty can only hold so many bricks before it will start to sink. To stay afloat, one must balance the amount of bricks and keep the floaty inflated.

In life, you will always have bricks, and what those bricks are will change throughout your life. It's your responsibility to monitor and make adjustments. You have to make sure you don't have so many bricks aboard that you sink. When you are feeling deflated, it's your responsibility to find the things that will get you pumped back up. Both factors are vital to staying afloat.

SAYING THANK YOU INSTEAD OF I'M SORRY

You should feel empowered to say no, but can you gracefully say no? How we say no matters.

My husband, Dakota, and I were just talking about the difference between saying thank you and saying I'm sorry. Dakota let me drop off Kennedy at his work on my way to an appointment. I mixed up the time of my appointment and dropped her off earlier than I needed to. I got stuck in my insecurity and kept messaging him how sorry I was for messing up his schedule. He was a champ and let her color while he finished working. I was so caught up in my insecurity that I kept apologizing instead of just telling him how much I appreciated him.

Apologizing too much can end up making the other person frustrated when they originally weren't. It's the constant apologizing, not the thing you're apologizing for, that can be frustrating. Can anyone else relate? I know I have this tendency.

This often happens when people say no. Instead of thanking the person for the opportunity, they become overwhelmed with guilt and keep apologizing.

If you treat someone like they're explosive, they will explode. I was treating Dakota like he should be frustrated with me. While looking for reassurance that he wasn't frustrated, I was treating him like he was.

Honestly, I am so proud of how far we've come. On the day this happened, we not only identified the patterns at play but talked through them in a matter of a few hours. It's times like these I see how much progress we've made.

If someone says no to my invitation, I would much rather they thank me for the opportunity than be apologetic. It shifts the whole vibe. I want the grateful, thankful, beautiful, "I am honored" vibes. When I say no, I love telling the other person I'm honored they thought of me. I am honored they would include me. When we use words like this, it builds people up. It assumes the best of them.

There is a time and place where apologies are appropriate. You should apologize if you committed to something you're no longer going to do. These instances should be rare.

Notice the difference in energy between apologizing and thanking. Compare the difference in facial expressions and body language. When you're thanking and complimenting, your body language will be happy, cheerful, thankful, and uplifting. Being thankful brings sunshine instead of clouds. When you're apologetic, your shoulders drop in, your head might tilt down, and your face will be low or frowning. It can be uncomfortable at first, but I challenge you to try thanking instead of apologizing.

Be clear and make your message positive. Create a path for them to have a positive response. Don't just hope they won't have a negative one. Believe the best about them and treat them accordingly.

HOW DO YOU EXPECT OTHERS TO TREAT YOU?

By asking for what you want, drawing relational boundaries, and saying no, you are teaching others how you want to be treated.

During this journey of transformational change, it can be tricky to catch your unwanted behavior upfront. It might be hard to see our thought patterns, negative influences, or relational patterns until it feels like we're too far in. As you practice, it will get clearer and easier to spot these things upfront. Don't be discouraged if you're seeing the same patterns over and over. Be encouraged you caught it sooner than last time.

If you don't do the work to recognize your patterns and take the necessary steps to change or break the cycle, you'll end up living with a lot of garbage you don't want in your life but feel helpless to change. A powerful way to break out of the victim mentality is to name your boundaries.

The purpose of this exercise is to bring to light some of your patterns and create a plan of action to weed them out of your life. Spend some time with these questions. No stinkin' thinkin' is permitted here. Think about yourself like royalty, as if you were a queen or king. Bring yourself to the highest standard and the most honored position. You may not feel like that now, but this is part of the process of feeling worthy. You define how you will be treated.

1. How do you want to be treated?
2. What are the behaviors you won't tolerate?
3. What are the steps you'll take to keep these behaviors out of your life?

Knowing how you expect to be treated gives you power. You can't stand firm on what you haven't established. I have found I can continue to refine and raise the bar as I get more comfortable standing up for myself. You'll build confidence and courage, and these things will become more natural as you keep setting limits for what you will allow in your life and what you will tolerate.

When you are setting boundaries, you can and should remain respectful and calm. By setting your boundaries before you even enter a situation, you'll help yourself keep firm and calm in the face of potential conflict. It's the same concept as an alarm clock. You aren't making the decision to wake up early when it is already morning. You've made the decision the night before, which makes it easier to stick to when your brain isn't fully engaged.

For me, setting boundaries began with not letting people raise their voices at me. As a child, I did not feel like I had the power to choose anything different for my life. It took me years into adulthood to figure out that I have the authority to say what I do and don't want in my life. I don't have to let people treat me a certain way. I can say no.

Start with finding one sentence and rehearse it over and over when you are alone. Anytime you think about the action you don't want in your life, boldly say your one sentence. In self-defense classes, they teach you that you'll freeze when you're in a dangerous situation, so you need to get the "freeze" out of the way. You practice your self-defense moves until it's muscle memory. In the same way, make your one sentence into muscle memory by repeating it out loud. This is a way to defend against being a victim.

One sentence I use is, "I reject what you just said." From the time my daughter was teeny-tiny, people thought they had the right to give their opinions without permission. I was shocked by the negativity people would project onto my daughter and our family.

I believe in the power of the spoken word. I'm especially passionate about it when it comes to my daughter, and even more so when she is standing right there.

Some might argue these boundaries don't always need to be said out loud. I have a few thoughts on that. If you're saying a boundary out loud but still internalizing your doubt, it won't do you any good to use your voice. On the flip side, saying them out loud can help you keep your doubt at bay. The more you claim your boundaries, whether externally or internally, the more confident you will become. Be firm in who you are and how you expect others to treat you.

When it comes to my daughter, I say my boundaries out loud for her as much as for me. Yes, it is my responsibility as a mom to reject the death spoken over my daughter. I also want my impressionable little human to see me defend and protect her and the beautiful, strong, amazing human God is growing her to be. I want to show her a graceful example of how to protect her spirit from the negative the world will try to project on her. I want her to know she has the authority to reject what is not hers to carry.

I hope that through my example, I can make a path for her to use her own voice. I will not always be there to fill the gap, but it's my job to be the example and pass her the reigns as she grows in strength and maturity. Sometimes, all I need to be is a gentle voice that says, "I believe more for you than that. You don't have to accept the voices of the world."

We teach our kids how to let others treat them by how we allow others to treat us. When they are little, they are looking to us to see if what is happening around them is okay. This happens even when they're only a couple of months old. This is huge. If we let other people tear us down, or the friends we hang out with are negative, they are watching. They are watching to see how we relate with others and how we care for others. They are watching our spoken and unspoken interactions. They're watching it all. They will be shaped by what you believe, whether you tell them what you believe or not.

Standing up for yourself does not have to tear anyone else down. It just lets other people know how serious you are about preserving and protecting your boundaries. The way I evaluate boundaries is by what is in my court. If there is a behavior I don't want in my life, I can't change the other person, but I can change my surroundings. Our boundaries are not up for debate. It isn't a discussion. It is powerful when you have enough confidence and belief in your worth to stand up and state your expectations. You can also set boundaries by removing yourself physically.

I want to acknowledge there are situations where you won't need to say anything, but your confidence will still shine through. When it is a pattern or ongoing cycle, you'll need to take action to change the trajectory. John Maxwell says in his book *15 Invaluable Laws of Growth*, "Remember, if you always do what you've always done, you'll always get what you've always gotten."[25] When there is an abusive pattern you've experienced your whole life, it will take a lot of work to stand up against it. This is why rehearsing is so valuable. Make a decision about how you will handle the situation before the boundary is crossed. Some situations will take more practice, more determination, and more grit than others.

---

[25] Maxwell, *The 15 Invaluable Laws of Growth*, 137.

<u>Chapter 7</u>

Be proactive in finding a positive community. Having others to turn to will help the path feel less lonely. It's easier to fall back into allowing toxic or abusive behavior if we don't have a support system. Be intentional about creating new relationships. Being in a group can sometimes make it easier to set your boundaries. It's easier to slip out of a conversation or change the direction of the conversation when you have support.

Through and through, you set the standard for how people treat you. For a long time, I thought I had to accept being treated poorly because of what I was getting in return—a job, help, friendship—but is that real friendship? At first, it might look like you're losing things left and right. Really, you're just refining your life. Sometimes, you have to let go of something to make room for a newer, better thing.

Believe you are worth it.

ACTION:

1. Do you have a question you are afraid to ask? What is holding you back?

2. In one conversation this week, voice that no is a valid answer when you are asking a question.

3. If you haven't already, answer these questions from the chapter:

    How do you want to be treated?

    What are the behaviors you won't tolerate?

    What are the steps you'll take to keep these behaviors out of your life?

4. What is the one sentence you can practice to set boundaries?

7

YOUR WORDS MATTER

I am a firm believer in the power of the spoken word. When I was discouraged about our home and our neighborhood, I found this verse, and it hit me hard. Proverbs 18:21 says, "The tongue can bring death or life."[26] I was claiming daily that our neighborhood didn't feel safe. I was saying that in front of my daughter and living in intense fear. Now, we live in the same place, and it is worlds apart based on the life I speak and pray over this neighborhood. Speaking life or death will shape your life.

One of the tricks I learned with kids was to always speak in a positive form. For example, when people say things to Kennedy like, "Don't trip," I say, "Keep your balance. You're doing great." By saying, "Don't trip," we shift our attention to the negative instead of the positive. Others might say, "She is being shy." We say, "She is being cautious, and cautious is wise." When someone points out, "That is hard," shift the focus and say, "That looks challenging, but you are a great problem solver." This applies just as much to adults. Instead of saying to a friend, "Don't forget your keys," say, "Remember your keys." Focus on where you want the focus to be, not the place you want to avoid.

When people chime in and give your child an excuse not to persevere or an out not to complete a task, these are the times I want to verbally affirm my child's capability. Can you see how asking a question like "Is that too hard?" and then doing the task for the kid wires their brain to give up? Yes, it is often easier to do the task yourself because it is quicker

---

[26] Proverbs 18:21 (New Living Translation).

and less messy. When we do that, are we shaping the kind of adult we want to raise?

I am such a proud mama when I hear my little lady correct her negative talk. The word "can't" is banned in our family, so when she catches herself and corrects it, it is so beautiful. She'll say, "I can do it, but would you help me this time?" or, "I think I could figure it out, but would you be willing to help me?"

I notice negative speaking patterns much more often when it is directed toward my daughter than when it is directed toward me. I stand in the gap when someone speaks death over my child. When someone projects their negative beliefs on my child, I take my authority and reject what they said. It's our job as parents to protect our children from the death spoken over them until they can learn how and discern it for themselves. Part of how they learn is by seeing it modeled for them.

Along the same lines, we can also thank our children for completing a task even if they haven't done it yet. If we are getting ready for bed, and I tell my daughter she needs to go to the shower, but she isn't listening, I might gently say, "Thank you for using your best obeying ears and heading straight to the shower." And a funny thing happens. She often does exactly what she is supposed to do.

Again, this applies to adults as well. We can thank our spouse for taking care of that thing that still needs to be done: "Thanks for being willing to take care of the grass. I really appreciate it." It has to be sincere. It has to come from a place of honest belief and thankfulness. You can be sincerely thankful they are willing to do something without it being done yet. A few years ago, I would have said these types of things out of frustration, not sincere thankfulness. If you're in the same boat, I'll tell you now it won't get the same results.

Mark Batterson writes in *The Circle Maker* about the faithfulness of praising before we see the results.[27] As hard as this can be sometimes, it makes so much sense. It is a way of speaking life.

One of my all-time favorite studies was done by IKEA. It was done with two plants, each in their own glass box, at a school. There were signs that told the students to talk kindly to one plant and unkindly to the other. The plant that was spoken to nicely thrived, and the one that was

---

[27] Batterson, *The Circle Maker*, 39–41.

spoken to rudely withered.[28] If this is true for plants, how much truer is it for humans? Speak life. It will create growth.

SAY YES AS OFTEN AS POSSIBLE

Kids hear the word "no" so much in their most formative years. I made it my mission to say yes as often as possible.

Even if the thing my daughter wants to do can't be done at that moment, I will still say yes. For example, if she wants to read a book, but we are playing at the park and have no books with us, I'll say, "Yes, we can read a book once we get home."

When she was in her toddler years and would ask the same question over and over again, we got well-practiced at asking back, "What is the answer?" It was easier for our daughter to wait when she knew the answer was yes. It is so affirming for her to say out loud that the answer is yes.

Another amazing tool is to reframe your statements with "When/ Then." For example, if someone says, "*If* you do your chores, *then* you can play with your toys," the child's behavior is then reliant on what they'll get in return. Reframing this statement as, "*When* you do your chores, *then* you can play with your toys," gives them the responsibility. You might also say, "When you get the dishes done, then you can play outside," or, "When you have cleaned your room, then you can have friends over."

The problem often isn't that we don't want to give our children what they're asking for. Playing outside and having friends over are positive things. The problem is often that the things we want them to get done, such as doing the dishes or cleaning their room, aren't getting done. When something like playing outside is framed as a reward, we as parents are the ones keeping them from the reward. When it's framed as their responsibility, they have to own their actions. We put up a wall when we could be building a bridge.

I want my communication to inspire and encourage my daughter, not frustrate and limit her. I know there will still be frustration, but ultimately, I am trying to point to an open door instead of making her feel trapped. I want my communication to be about what *can be done*, not what can't.

---

[28] IKEA UAE, "Bully a Plant: Say No to Bullying," YouTube, April 30, 2018, video, 2:17, https://www.youtube.com/watch?v=Yx6UgfQreYY.

TAKE RESPONSIBILITY FOR YOUR FEELINGS

Have you ever heard a parent or teacher say to a child, "You're not going to like that," when the child wants to try something new? This doesn't happen only in childhood. People will try to tell us how we feel our whole lives. Sometimes it's subtle, and sometimes it's more obvious, but it's all manipulation.

There's a difference between asking someone how they feel and *telling* them how they feel. For example, you could ask a child, "Did that scare you?" instead of asking, "That was scary, huh?" We could ask, "Did that hurt?" instead of being quick to say, "That hurt, didn't it?" We could even take one more step back and ask, "How did that make you feel?" Try to ask open-ended questions that give people the space to say their real answers.

When we are too quick to label someone's feelings, we write their story for them. Being too quick to label someone else's experience can cause them to shut down and mistrust themselves. It can be invalidating. Think of how confusing and flustering it is when we don't have the right words and people keep interjecting their descriptions. It isn't what you want to say, but you stop correcting them. It can leave people feeling unheard.

One of the most vivid examples of this I have was this time my daughter, who was about one and a half at the time, wanted to play with my coworker's basketball. When she asked if she could play with it, he told her, "You don't want that. It's dirty." Instead of telling her no and redirecting her or finding something else she could play with, he told her, "You don't want that." That is directly contradicting what her little mind is computing. Over time, this can cause a person to second-guess and stop trusting themself.

When people say things like, "Don't go in the puddle. You don't want to get dirty," that is the person pawning off what *they* want. Their motivation is probably not wanting to argue or face their own discomfort with being direct and holding boundaries. People do this simply because they are trying to avoid conflict. It is easier for them to speak in a nice, sweet voice and tell us *we* don't want something. If we take the bait, confrontation is avoided.

On the surface, this can seem harmless. The problem is, if the child is pursuing the puddle, they probably don't mind being dirty. In my view, the strategy might work for now, but it is setting the stage for future problems. It is creating codependency. It is setting the stage for rebellion. What happens when the kid finally does stand up and says, "That isn't what I think. That is what you think." They will figure it out one day, and when they do, there will likely be resentment.

It is so positive to allow kids to think for themselves within clear boundaries. When we resist, we take something away from them and hinder the relationship. We can still be a part of the decision-making process and have influence, but we shouldn't tell our children how they feel. This isn't allowing the child to have their own thoughts and opinions. It's healthier to tell them, "Mommy doesn't want you to get wet right now, so no going in the puddle." It might feel funny and more demanding than you want to sound, but you'll be separating what is in your court and what is in theirs. You can even acknowledge their desire when they persist: "I hear that you want to go in the puddle." Even though they aren't getting the answer they want, being heard offers safety and connection. This is so valuable, especially in their developing years.

The most important thing is to be clear. I'm going to continue with the puddle example. What are the parameters? Express them directly. Maybe you say, "You can jump in the puddle, but I'm not changing your clothes until we get home. You might get cold, but that is your choice."

So many people with good intentions are trying to protect their children from being uncomfortable or getting hurt, but in doing so, they are actually taking away opportunities to build trust. Don't change the boundary halfway through. If you said, "It's not okay today," then stick with it, but if there are any choices you can let your child make, let them make them.

When I nannied, I had one little guy under the age of two who was so confident physically. While I was still learning his ability level, I would stay near him and see what he could do while being ready to save him from injury. He never failed to surprise me with his level of skill. Kids will find their limits if we let them. Adults often hold them back.

One of the best things I ever did with kids I nannied was to let them fall. It builds trust. I broke their fall at the bottom so they didn't hit the ground too hard, but I let them experience the feeling of falling. I let them get up on their own, and I was right there to brush them off. I was there to affirm whatever feelings they were having. I didn't try to convince them that it was scary; I just let them have the experience safely and was present to comfort them. They will learn quickly with experience.

Sometimes, we need to let them have the experience they think they want so badly. If we try to convince them not to do something, it will be an ongoing battle. Oftentimes, they'll find out for themselves it isn't what they thought it would be. They just need the closure of testing it for themselves. We'll still be right there for them, and letting them have the experience and being a safe place for them to come back to builds trust.

If we can teach them in a controlled environment, then they find their limits and know they can trust you. Over time, with small experiences, they may be less inclined to test for themselves what you advise against because they trust in you. Once they associate your suggestions with protecting them and not limiting them, they will be more willing to listen.

Instead of telling them not to do something, try telling them what the consequence might be and allowing them to choose if they'd like to proceed. Once they experience firsthand that being cold makes them shiver, they can decide if the fun is worth the consequences. Maybe what would be a no for you is a yes for them. That's okay.

If your child asks you if they can do something and your answer is no, that is okay too. Remember, it is kinder to say no and be clear than to try and put your feelings on them. In our family, if bad attitudes arise when the answer is no, we redirect to thankfulness. When our daughter isn't handling the answer no well, we tell her how thankful we are for all the things we did get to do and the time we spent doing it. It's a beautiful thing to see the attitude shift. This might not happen every time, but it is a great tool to have in your tool belt. This practice is good for me too. When I direct my attention to gratefulness, I am better able to empathize with her feelings and be patient.

The way we speak shapes our lives. Be intentional, observant, and thoughtful about how you are investing.

YOU'RE GIVING ME LIFE

How often do we hear the phrase "you're killing me" in reference to something that is making us so happy we can't contain it? My daughter and her daddy are so cute together. When I watched them play, I started catching myself saying, "You're killing me," but that is the opposite of what it is doing. I quickly changed my saying to, "You're giving me life!" It brings so much light and life and joy to see them together doing their thing, laughing, and playing. I want my expression of joy to bring light and life too.

We have so many little sayings in our culture that are habitual. They don't bring life, but we excuse them with, "You know what I mean." That's not the point. Our culture is saturated with thoughtless and negative forms of communication. They're normal because they haven't been challenged. You can have more light and life in your life by making simple, attainable shifts in your language. We often get caught up in thinking we need some huge life-altering experience to change our lives. I am here to tell you that isn't true. It is the small things. Start being intentional about the seemingly insignificant, excusable, habitual language in your life that is speaking death, not life.

Some people might view this as picky and ridicule your obsessiveness, but this is an example of people who are willing to drag you down with them. Over time, your life will be so drastically different that it will be worth it.

BELIEVE IN YOURSELF FOR THEM

I am strong in mind and body.
I have authority over my body.
I am incredible.
I am valuable.
I am a daughter of the King.
Jesus loves me.
And so does Mommy.
And so does Daddy.

I've been saying these affirmations with Kennedy from the time she could talk. The list has grown as time has gone on, and the list of who loves her and who is on her mind that night extends far and wide. I embrace it because I want her to know how loved she is. I am thankful she knows so many people love her. Before you say it, I know she's procrastinating bedtime and keeping me as long as she can, but man, I have come to treasure this time.

There was a point where I was struggling with my confidence and not speaking life for myself. During that time, Kennedy refused to do the affirmations. This broke my heart. I want more than anything for her to see her value. I want her to believe in herself and know how much she is treasured and loved. I want her to know that she is unstoppable.

Through this season, I saw how important it was for me to believe in myself for her. When she sees me believe in myself, she starts to believe in herself. You can't fake it with kids. From a young age, they pick up on what you believe about yourself. We can tell them all the positive things in the world, but they are picking up on our actions and our words, what we accept from others, and how we treat ourselves. If those things aren't lining up, there is a disconnect.

This feels so close to my heart because my dad made the effort to give us kids all the positive beliefs that no one gave him. He wanted us to have the beliefs that he didn't have for himself. My dad was saying the right words, but there was still a void, a gap. He wanted to foster in us a belief in ourselves, but he didn't have the foundation to do it. To me, it's like the feeling of having a word on the tip of your tongue, but you can't quite figure it out. It's elusive.

When Kennedy wouldn't say the affirmations, it made me so sad. I could feel the divide between trying to throw all the right tools her way and not living it for myself. She wasn't buying it. I wanted it for her so badly. I had to do more than want it for her. I had to fight for me, for her. I had to show her I believed it as well.

We won't ever have it all figured out. There will always be obstacles we can't foresee. That is the beautiful thing about a firm foundation—you don't have to have it all figured out. If you have a strong sense of identity and security, each obstacle will have less weight. When we model this for our kids, it gives them strength. It is modeling the power we are speaking in and over them. They can identify with the strength because they feel it exuding out of you.

It's not an elusive concept. They know exactly what it feels like, and they can build on it.

WILL YOU LET ME KNOW EITHER WAY?

I used to feel so trapped by communication, or the lack of it. My programming told me to walk on eggshells and not offend anyone. I felt subject to whatever others did or didn't say. I'd be waiting for a response to a question, and often people wouldn't know I was still waiting. They'd think they'd answered already or wouldn't realize there was a question to answer. In my desire not to frustrate anyone, I wouldn't assert myself.

I've found so much power in having simple one-line phrases that are clear and direct. One of these phrases is, "Will you let me know either way?" This states I am looking for an answer. This gives them the freedom to say no or ask what the question is.

I have learned to bring clarity and authority to what I am saying. Even if being direct is uncomfortable, it is more kind than being unclear. This reminds me of the saying from Brené Brown: "Clear is kind. Unclear is unkind."[29] We live in a culture where people want the truth sugarcoated. A common excuse I hear is, "I don't want to sound mean."

You don't have to be mean to say the truth, and saying the truth isn't mean.

SAYING NEGATIVE QUALITIES
IN THE PAST TENSE

I love the practice of only saying negative qualities in the past tense. It doesn't have to be referring to something in the distant past. It could be a negative action from yesterday. That is still in the past, and today will be better.

Speaking about our struggles in this way keeps us from claiming negativity for our lives or putting limits on our growth. It allows us to claim the positive we want and work toward it.

It takes time to make this a regular practice. Start with noticing when you're talking about negative qualities in the present tense. Maybe you say, "I have a bad temper." When we claim these qualities in the present tense,

---

[29] Brené Brown, "Clear Is Kind. Unclear Is Unkind." *Brené Brown*, October 15, 2018, https://brenebrown.com/articles/2018/10/15/clear-is-kind-unclear-is-unkind. <u>Chapter 8</u>

we are reinforcing the negative and making it even harder to change. Start switching your mindset and say instead, "In the past, I have had a bad temper, but I am working on it."

This is a small shift in speech but a huge leap for your brain. Tell your brain that today is a new day, and you have the chance to be the best version of yourself today. This gives us a fighting chance to not bring yesterday's failures into today. Soon we won't bring them into the next week, the next month, and then the next year.

We all have a story. We are all overcomers. We are all on a journey. When other people can experience your imperfection without the burden of needing to figure out what to do with it, they can just be encouraged by your story.

I faced severe depression during my pregnancy with my daughter. After I climbed out of that deep pit, I thought it would never happen again. My husband and I were in the middle of such extreme circumstances when it happened, so I thought the depression must be a one-time thing. It took me off guard when I faced it again. After recovering the second time, I began to be fearful and anticipate it coming again. In this way, I gave it power over my life.

By speaking in the past tense about my depression, I could frame it differently. It was something I had overcome multiple times. Instead of seeing it as a possibility for my future, it became a thing of the past. I am not leaving room for it to be an option in my present or future.

Putting our struggles in the past helps us make a change today. It makes today a new start. When we're intentional about saying our negative qualities in the past tense, we give ourselves a fighting chance to be a better version of ourselves. Our brains need us to stop carrying the old baggage so we can become the new self.

ACTION:

1. Identify a situation in your life when you tend to speak in the negative form. How can you change your language and speak in the positive form?

2. What is one common phrase you use that is speaking death instead of life? How can you change that phrase to speak life?

3. Identify some of the things that keep you from being clear. What's one phrase you can use to be clear?

4. What's one quality you can start speaking about in the past tense?

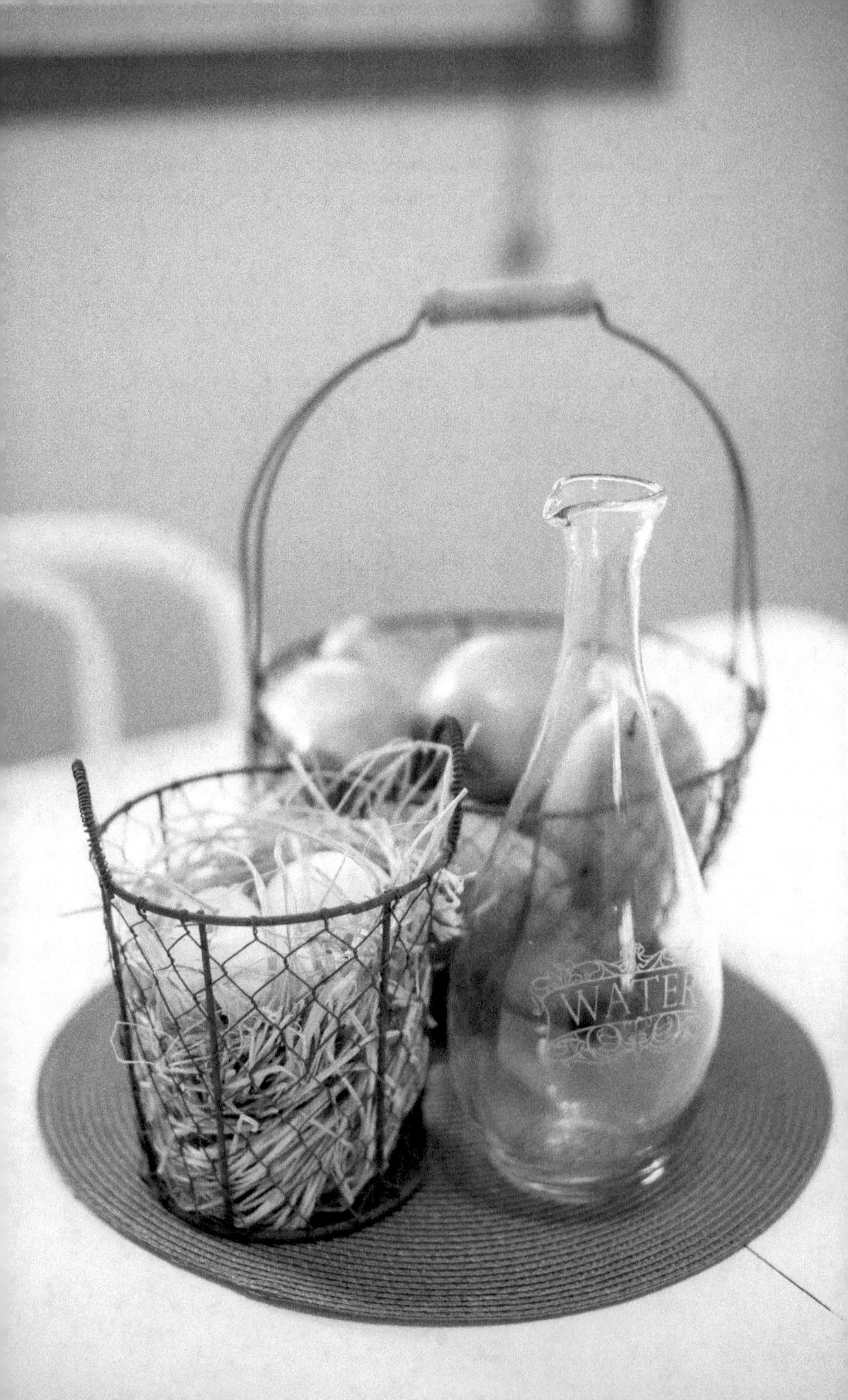

WATER

PART 3

WHOLE-BODY HEALTH

8

TAKING CARE OF YOUR MENTAL HEALTH

When I first began writing this book, I was so structured about when I would sit down to write. As I got further along, I went through phases where I resisted sitting down to work. I tried to make it easier by pampering myself before writing. I would take a shower, use scented lotion, make tea, and light a candle. These were the things that made me feel calm and prepared me to just be.

One night, after I got my daughter down and was prepping, I caught myself having the thought, "I don't have time to take care of myself this much every night." That hit me hard. Why shouldn't I take the time to take care of myself? God taught me so many lessons through my season of rest, and this was a big one.

I have a hard time treating myself. I'll find myself getting mad and frustrated at my body for what it needs. I've found that I need more sleep than most people. By contrast, my husband needs way less sleep than the average person. This makes me feel like I am *always* sleeping. I do so much better when I just listen to my body and give it what it needs.

When your body is asking something of you, instead of rejecting it, find a way you can enjoy giving it what it needs. Some people naturally need to exercise more, and some naturally have to be more restrictive with their diet or like me, sleep. The more I embrace this and schedule around my needs, the more efficient I am with the time I have. Then I can do what's really important.

One of the misconceptions about self-care is the amount of time it takes or how expensive it can be. Self-care can start with a handful of

91

small things that take half an hour or less and cost twenty dollars or less. I have found it's more effective to have little things on a regular basis rather than one extravagant activity. Make a routine that feels like a treat, even if it's simple.

Having a clean house is one of the most peaceful feelings for me, so I maximize that. My husband and I clean the house after our little one is down on Thursday nights. Once the house is done, I shower, get snuggly, get the diffuser going, and often I have a little treat. Most of these nights include sitting on the couch with a new book I haven't flipped through yet. This can take an hour or less and is so refreshing. This feels like pampering to me.

REFRESHING YOUR SOUL

When I say refreshing your soul, I mean truly replenishing it, not just coping. As I told you earlier, food has been one of my drugs, and I didn't even know it until I took my year of rest. I knew working was one of the ways I coped, but I didn't realize how much I depended on it until I set it down for my year of rest. It's only when I didn't have it that I could see how often I turned to it. These types of unhealthy coping mechanisms aren't the things that will replenish and refresh you. They may make you more comfortable temporarily, but they aren't truly replenishing. The key is finding the things that give you true rest and recovery.

Let's use TV as an example. A lot of people are in denial about how they use TV for coping or running. A lot of people use TV to check out. It isn't replenishing them. They are just hiding or avoiding their problems. I'm not saying all TV is bad, but bring awareness to how, when, and why you are watching it.

I am very protective of what I watch. I have a very sensitive spirit and know I have to be careful of what I allow into my mind. With that being said, over the years I have found a few shows that help me process life and put words to things I couldn't before. Honest to goodness, some of my biggest breakthroughs have come from watching a show. Somehow, watching a character process their life brings out the things that have been tucked away in my own life. Maybe I didn't realize I needed healing, but when I can relate to a character and their struggles, seeing their progress can help me decide my next step. Sometimes, they even come to a conclusion or revelation I needed.

A friend once told me if there is ever a movie that makes you cry, watch it again and keep watching it until you figure out why it makes you cry. The same concept comes up in John Eldredge's book *Get Your Life Back*. He says that if something moves you or makes you cry, God may be using it as a tool for healing. He says to name the feelings behind it, embrace the memories, bring God in, and allow the healing.[30]

Earlier in this book, I asked you to evaluate what it is you run to and use as unhealthy coping mechanisms. Now I want you to think deeply about what replenishes your soul.

WHAT YOU TELL YOURSELF

What you tell yourself during the morning and night can change the trajectory of your days.

I went through a phase where I would roll out of bed, look out the window, and actually notice what my first thought of the day was. All too often, we just let those thoughts happen. The course of my days used to be determined by things that were out of my control: it would be a good day if the sunshine was out when I woke up, but I'd be mad if it was dark when I woke up. Now I choose how my day will go by being intentional with how I speak to myself first thing in the morning.

I do well with structure, goals, and lists. Sometimes at night, if I don't have a clear direction for the following day, my mind starts to feel chaotic. Without clear direction, I can subconsciously decide it will be a disorganized, sluggish, or unproductive day. The change is so subtle I wouldn't realize I was making that decision. This is an example of not taking charge of my thoughts.

I have found that declaring, "I am excited for tomorrow," helps me look forward to what is to come. I can feel good about my day without having to compulsively rehearse what the day will bring. I rest in the thought that tomorrow will be good. Whether that day will bring chores or fun, I am excited.

---

[30] John Eldredge, *Get Your Life Back: Everyday Practices for a World Gone Mad* (Nashville: Thomas Nelson, 2020).

This has been a valuable practice for me, especially when I have had a hard day. I sometimes want to go to bed cranky and hope I magically wake up feeling better. Don't get me wrong, sometimes sleep is what we need to feel better, but we choose to feed our brains good or bad.

Begin to notice what thoughts you are having at the beginning and end of the day. Be intentional about what you choose for your days. Here are some phrases you can say with intention in the morning:

- Today will be a good day.
- I am excited for today.
- I am thankful for today.
- I choose to love and be loved today.
- Today is a beautiful day.
- Today is an incredible day to be alive.

Here are some phrases you can say with intention at night:

- Tomorrow holds so much opportunity.
- I am excited for tomorrow.
- I will make the most of tomorrow.
- I will make healthy choices tomorrow.
- I will find the beauty in tomorrow.
- Tomorrow is going to be a good day.
- Tomorrow is another opportunity to grow.
- Tomorrow is a turning point.

WORK OUT FOR YOUR MIND

I ran competitively for years. I ran during all of middle school and high school and during one year of college. I took it very seriously, and especially in high school, it was my lifeline. I got an injury a few years ago that prevents me from running now, but I still know I do better when I exercise.

I was intrigued by the results a friend of mine got from doing thirty-minute at-home workouts. I committed to working out for thirty minutes three days a week. The first week, I found myself thinking, "Work out for your mind if not for your body."

My mind needs me to work out my body. My mind needs my body to stick to its commitment and push itself. Physical exercise is connected so strongly to our mental health. It not only makes you stronger physically, but it builds confidence and makes you stronger mentally. I am training my mind to be strong by helping my body be strong. When I was running, my coaches always said running is a mental sport. Exercise is about mental toughness. It is about discipline. It's about doing what you said you were going to do.

I loved running for my high school team. I loved my teammates and my coaches. I loved the high. I loved how I felt after a really hard workout. I loved ultimate frisbee workouts. Most of all, I loved who I saw in the mirror. I saw a strong, capable, hardworking, achieving, positive, energetic, barrier-breaking, goal-setting, confident person.

These are my most important tips for working out:

1. Make a commitment to yourself, not just a wish.
2. Make it a routine.
3. Remember your "why."

<u>Make a commitment to yourself, not just a wish:</u>

Working out doesn't just happen. You can't just make a wish and get the results you want. My husband and I moved every year for the first six years of our marriage. Every time we moved, I had to find a new exercise routine. That would take time, and then we would move again. I was off and on with exercise for years. It is difficult even when you stay in one place. The seasons change, it gets dark sooner or later, some days there is snow on the ground, and our little human has different needs as she gets older. It takes persistence to keep exercise in my routine.

Make a commitment to yourself. Maybe you need to start small. Commit to thirty minutes three days a week. Schedule those times into your calendar so they don't just slip by. And guess what? If it is 10:00 p.m. on a Sunday night and you remember you haven't worked out at all this week, make yourself work out for an hour and a half. Do it! I am telling you, don't let yourself get off the hook with any excuses.

I came up with a very extreme business strategy, so try to go with it for a minute. What if when you signed up for a gym, you told them how much time you want to spend working out? As long as you hold that commitment, the gym is free. The catch is you have to pay a fee, let's say $10, if you miss your workout. Another way to do this would be you pay the gym at the beginning of the month, and every time you work out, they pay you back. (Someone should totally put these ideas into action and tell me how it goes.)

When there are no tangible and immediate consequences, it's too easy to skip. There are all kinds of positive effects of working out, which means there are negative consequences to not working out. So get serious about making a commitment to yourself, whatever that takes. Maybe you make yourself pay money if you miss a workout. You could tithe the money, give it to a mission, drop it on the ground, or whatever works for you. Maybe you could put it in a jar and pick who or what that money will be supporting at the end of the month. Whatever you choose, do it immediately when you have missed or chosen not to do the workout. Feel the discomfort of not sticking to your commitment. Writer and entrepreneur Jim Rohn said, "We must all suffer one of two things: the pain of discipline or the pain of regret."[31]

If money motivates you, maybe "pay" yourself to work out. I'm suggesting this idea because I 100% think you do not need a gym. Look up how much a gym would cost per month and figure out how much that cost would be per week or workout. Every time you stick to your commitment, you get paid. Now the money you would be willing to spend on working out is just a reward. I say that's a double win.

When I was running, I learned that sometimes the days when you least want to run turn out to be the best days to run. That's why it is so important to do it even when you don't feel like it. When you get done, take that deep inhale and feel the satisfaction of a job well done. You'll be so glad you decided to run. And it will be easier to do the next time you think you don't want to. Keep your commitment to yourself.

<u>Make it a routine:</u>

---

[31] "10 Unforgettable Quotes by Jim Rohn," *SUCCESS*, September 17, 2019, https://www.success.com/10-unforgettable-quotes-by-jim-rohn/.
<u>Chapter 11</u>

I love working out first thing in the morning. It is one of those things that builds a strong foundation for the day and helps keep balance and perspective. I have gone through different seasons with different routines. I went through a season of exercising when Kennedy went down for a nap. Doing a thirty-minute workout at the beginning of naptime ensures I won't run out of time, even if she wakes up early or a project takes longer than I thought. It actually makes it feel like I have more time. Thirty minutes can feel like a whole two hours some days, so when I still have three-fourths of the time left, I am pleased.

It doesn't matter when you choose to work out. Being consistent is the key. Being consistent helps your body get in a rhythm and will make you more likely to remember to work out. Eventually, your body will start craving the exercise.

<u>Remember your "why":</u>

I want to challenge you to make a list of what motivates you to work out. It's so easy to forget why we do these things for ourselves. Is it so your kids can see you healthy and strong? Is it so you stay fit for your spouse? Is it for your overall health? So you can build confidence and positive thoughts about yourself? Is it so you can be around for your great-grandkids? The list can be wide and deep.

Why is exercising important to you? Narrow this down to something you can put on a sticky note on your bathroom mirror. On the days you don't feel like exercising, you can look at your note and see the bigger purpose.

Then, make another list that shows how you want to feel about yourself. Being a former athlete, it's like I can go back into those feelings, especially when I breathe in the crisp fall air. The fall breeze evokes memories of the cross country season. It takes me back to the feelings of rest, contentment, satisfaction, and achievement I felt when I ran. I will close my eyes, breathe in deeply, and just soak up those good feelings. It's something that helps me be 100% Ame. It makes my soul feel whole.

Maybe you weren't an athlete, but there was something, maybe baking with your grandma, swimming, dancing, anything that gave you those strong feelings of security, identity, and strength. What are those things you wish you felt about yourself now? Exercise can help you come back to those feelings. Fight for that.

MAKE SMALL ADJUSTMENTS

In Part 1 of this book, we discussed how we can't rush and force our way through our journeys of healing. I have found this is also true for our mental health.

In the seasons when I have been fighting depression, I have had to learn to open my hands and release my judgment and frustration. Instead of holding my fists tight and trying to battle it in the boxing ring, I need to acknowledge and honor it. It is wild how much more quickly my depression seems to evaporate when I don't try to beat it and when I don't beat myself up for being where I am. I still have to do the work to get out of the pit, but at least I'm not digging myself in deeper.

Sometimes on windy days, my dad would take me and my siblings to the park down the road, cheap kites in hand. When I would get my kite into the air, I would run around the field, periodically looking back to make sure it was still in the air. When the tension on the string broke, I would turn toward the kite and use my whole body to pull and tug at it, trying desperately to keep it in the air. When the kite did crash, I would wind the string back up and throw it back into the air. When I was sure I had control over it, I would let it out a few feet at a time and make sure it was steady.

This is how depression feels to me. I'll let the string of my life go out farther than I can manage, and it comes crashing down. This happens when I am pushing too hard, forgetting to rest, and losing track of where my true value comes from. I have to reel everything back in and start over with a short string. Then I let it out a few feet at a time.

The thing is, I want to stop crashing the kite. I am figuring out what distance I can let the kite out before I begin to lose control. I need to keep the distance in a manageable place so, if I start to lose control, I can reel it in a little. On the other hand, when it is steady, I can give a little slack. I can make the adjustment that needs to be made without losing control and crashing.

This is why rest and balance are so important to our lives. One of the main things that has helped me is keeping a routine that makes room for the things that restore and replenish me. When I am starting to feel out of control, I have to slow down and remind myself of the things that God has taught me through my year of rest.

Overcoming a hurdle like depression can feel overwhelming, so just start with the small steps. I have such a clear memory of this friend who used to drive me home from school on occasion. When we got off the main roads, they would let me steer the car from the passenger seat. Every time the car started drifting to one side just a little, I would overcorrect and jerk the wheel back to the other side. My friend gave me gentle advice that applies to so much more than just driving. They said, "Make small adjustments." Seriously, this advice has applied to so many situations in my life. I have a tendency to overcorrect and often have to remind myself it might just need a little tweaking.

You don't have to change every aspect of your life. Oftentimes, you just need to add or subtract a few key habits. It all starts with small, steady adjustments.

ACTION:

1. Find a handful of simple activities that make you feel like you have taken extra care of yourself and implement them each once a week.

2. Create an exercise routine by answering the questions:

    What are your top three forms of exercise?

    What time of day works best for you to exercise?

    How many days a week are you going to do a thirty-minute (or longer) workout?

3. Can you tell when there is too much slack in your life? When do you need to reel it in before everything crashes?

4. What are three small adjustments you can make that would have a positive impact?

9

TAKING CARE OF YOUR PHYSICAL HEALTH

Ever since I competed in high school cross country, I have been interested in whole-body health, but it was only in my year of rest that I got serious about applying the concepts and theories to my life. I have learned a ton about my body and how to respect what it is trying to communicate. I got to a point where I could no longer keep my health at the bottom of the list. I had to make it a priority.

This intentionality has been rewarded with my days feeling longer and fuller. Exercising doesn't deplete my energy—it gives me more of it. I feel healthier and more vibrant when I eat the foods that fit my blood type and have the self-control to stop eating when I am full. I am so excited to share what I've been learning, and I hope something I say sparks you to make changes for a healthier future.

I have been on an incredible food journey. It all started when I got a rash on my face that just kept spreading. I put everything on it I could think of. It got to the point where I could hardly open my mouth to eat. At first, the skin irritation spread slowly. Then overnight, it became unbearable. That's when I started calling naturopathic doctors' offices all around town to see who could get me in immediately.

I began working with a naturopathic doctor to assess what was happening in my body. I needed to know what my body was trying to communicate. Long story short, I began the process of healing my gut. I didn't understand all the big words they used, but the basic idea was that my stomach wasn't doing its job. I had not been taking good care of it. I discovered I had poor food hygiene, and that was only the beginning of the discovery.

After my second session with my new doctor, I went home with a list of nutrients that needed to be added back into my body. The period between my second and third appointments was dreadfully painful. My doctor had recommended using the basics of the Paleo diet to guide my food choices. I jumped in and changed my diet completely. I am much more comfortable with black-and-white directions, so having a diet to reference felt safe to me. Even if it was going to be a hard or drastic shift, I needed the boundaries. I committed to the Paleo diet till my next appointment.

I had such high hopes that if I could just figure out what to feed my body, we could get along. I needed some hope that whatever was going on it could be handled naturally. Instead, I felt out of control, angry, and irritable. I fought depression and being so eerily tired that it brought on more depression.

After more time and more appointments, I learned that healing my gut was as much about my relationship with food as it was about what I ate. I wanted a list of what foods I could eat endlessly and what was off-limits. I can follow that. I had to learn that this was a journey about listening to my body, not a black-and-white list.

I found that my relationship with food was a sour one. A lot of the problems I was having stemmed from overeating. This was a monumental realization for me. That was when I was able to verbalize that I grew up with food insecurity. This helped me learn to listen to my body.

I had been eating out of insecurity. I ran to sugar when I didn't feel like I had a voice. My go-to comfort was a can of frosting in the cupboard. I have never struggled with my weight, so a lot of my food issues stayed in their secret closet. There wasn't a physical sign that something needed to change. That was until a skin irritation appeared that couldn't be covered or hidden.

The interesting thing about my naturopathic doctor's instructions was he was simply helping my body do what it was made to do. He gave me some practical exercises for practicing good food hygiene. It was gentle suggestions, not demands. Someone once told me your body will naturally sigh when it's full. It might not seem like we are full, but this is our body's subtle way of letting us know to stop eating. I began to notice that sigh more often, and even if I didn't stop eating, I would at least try to listen to it. I would put my utensils down. Then I got to where I would push my dish away. As I listened to my body's signals and started testing them, I found I could trust them.

The timing of my skin irritation seems kind of wild if you don't believe in a God with perfect timing. It began about a month after I committed to taking a year of rest. Just a couple of months later, I began to suspect that maybe it was caused by something emotional, not just physical. A lot of emotional things were bubbling to the surface that I didn't have the proper tools to cope with. I was not only committed to not taking my drug of working, but I was facing some really tough stuff as I began working with a counselor trained in EMDR, or eye movement desensitization and reprocessing. My body was at a breaking point. It needed intervention and insight from someone trained in listening to what the body is saying.

I honestly don't think I could have gone through this journey without a professional guiding me through it. When I got to my third meeting with my naturopathic doctor, he explained the out-of-control, angry, irritable, depressed feelings I had been having after meeting two were symptoms of "disrupting the numbing pattern." I was experiencing turbulence because I was removing the destructive pattern of overeating from my life. I was removing the pattern that had been instilled in me by my childhood.

He said, "Just because you were nurtured by that doesn't mean you will become that." That can apply to whatever your struggle is. If you have a negative pattern in your life that came from the way you were raised, you don't have to accept that pattern. You can change it.

I walked out of the doctor's office feeling like a new person. I had known I was going to take this health and food journey seriously, but the revelations that come from it can still knock me off my feet. Sometimes it feels like I was knocked into a lake and forgot how to swim, but coming out of those meetings reminds me of my reasons for doing this and my strength. I want to heal my body, live empowered, provide more stability for my daughter, and be the best version of myself. This makes it worth the work for me.

Our emotional and physical health are woven so tightly together. That is the value of whole-body care. We live in a culture that tries to separate the emotional from the physical, and it is only making us sicker.

Jesus wants your whole self. When we live in the light of Christ and let it illuminate every aspect of our being, there can be health and balance.

NATURAL MEDICINE

I believe God gave us everything in nature to balance and heal our bodies. What our culture calls alternative medicine is the medicine God gave us. I'd like to challenge the mindset of being doomed to accept a diagnosis even if a medical doctor doesn't know what's causing your symptoms. I am not discounting that specialized medical doctors have their place, but my experience is that the deeper answers are more likely to be solved with a broader evaluation of your life.

I especially want to challenge the idea that if it isn't modern medicine, it isn't of God. Here is where you need to use discernment and judgment. If you are walking in a relationship with God, ask Him for guidance.

In the past, when I would have a conviction from God, I would consult my Christian friends before deciding whether to act on it and then make my decision based on what they said. I would end up living in a pile of guilt because I wasn't living in alignment with my convictions. Be confident in where the Lord is leading you. You don't have to live in fear over what others think, even other Christians who are living differently than you.

I am not a medical professional. I want to share my experiences and tell you about the benefits I have found in natural medicine. I know what the line is for me, and that is an ongoing conversation in my spiritual journey. I encourage you to do the same thing. Do your research and talk to people you trust who work in healthcare. Ask them their "why." Talk to God about it. Don't just take my word for it.

God gave everything a purpose. The more I learn, the more amazed I am by the profound benefits of plants across the board. The benefits of eating them, using them for disease, and using them in place of over-the-counter medicine stretch far and wide. Our culture is far removed from nature and what can be grown, often in your own yard, for medicine. I'm not talking about plants that have to be grown to a certain maturity or cooked a certain way so they aren't harmful. I'm talking about basic plants, herbs, and weeds. Something as simple as smelling the rosemary in my garden can help clear my sinuses.

Just this morning (this goes to show how new I am to gardening), I found a cluster of bulbs that had been in the ground for years. A few weeks ago, my husband and I were wondering if bulbs come back every year and how you get more. As I was splitting this clump of dirt and looking at the bulbs, I realized they were like garlic. The bulbs are how they reproduce. I was fascinated by how simple and complex it is all at the same time. There is someone out there laughing at this because it is something you learned as a young child gardening with your mother or grandma. My daughter will be in the same boat as you, but my experience is common.

Using natural resources has helped dramatically with my sleep. I used to have nightmares. I couldn't make it through the night without shaking my husband awake. At the time, I didn't know anything about the benefits of Himalayan salt lamps. We happened to get one to use as a soothing night light. A few weeks went by before I realized I hadn't had any nightmares recently. Later, I found out that this kind of rock changes negative energy waves into positive ones. Years later, I still sleep with a salt lamp. I still occasionally have nightmares, but nothing like what it was.

I had an incredibly positive experience with magnet therapy. It helped me be able to breathe deeply when my sinuses were congested. The gal who worked with me was a Christian and prayed over me after our session. It was an incredibly healing experience. This is an example of someone living in their strength. This woman used her knowledge while working in the Spirit of God. God gives us so much insight into our body from science. Things like massage, reflexology, muscle testing, magnet therapy, and acupuncture can tell us so much about what is happening in our bodies. Using these tools can highlight what needs attention and even recenter our bodies.

There are a lot of professionals working in natural medicine that are not faith-based. I think this is why the Christian community can be so harsh and turn completely away from natural approaches. The interesting thing is this is also true in the world of modern medicine. There are Christian and non-Christian professionals on both sides. I have worked with some people I won't go back to because of this, but there are many people who don't impose their beliefs or non-beliefs and can use their expert knowledge without planting seeds of doubt. No matter who you work with, it is important to use discernment and guard your spirit.

In my experience, people who are educated in natural medicine are more focused on whole-body health and the effects of your environment. They don't just cover up your symptoms—they get to the root. Throughout my life, I have gotten breakouts on my hands. They cause my hands to get so cracked they bleed. These breakouts followed me into adulthood, and I reluctantly went to see a dermatologist. I wanted an answer about why this was happening, not a bandage. I didn't know where to turn. When I went into the office, the doctor diagnosed me in thirty seconds. He didn't have an explanation for the breakouts and just gave me a prescription for a steroid cream, then sent me on my way. I cried. I was so discouraged because this didn't feel like an answer to me.

It wasn't until I began seeing a naturopathic doctor for the rash on my face that I was willing to ask about this reoccurring skin issue again. The naturopathic doctor answered all my questions and was able to get to the root of the issue. I felt so much relief when I received a deeper, purposeful answer. I could solve the problem instead of just treating the symptoms.

Our world is in a health crisis no matter how you choose to deal with the symptoms. Instead of changing their lifestyle and habits, practicing self-control, and working on the root of the issue, people are settling for surface resolutions. After going through this process and this journey, I can admit I have gotten frustrated and even angry at times seeing so many people take the easy way out. The work is hard, and it will be an upheaval of your comfort, but it is real change. It is our responsibility to tune into our bodies and learn from and about them. There is lasting healing when we dig to the roots.

I am 100% pro-natural medicine and see how God is at work through it. He made our bodies so intricate and designed them to communicate with us. They'll tell us what we need to know to keep them healthy if only we will listen.

HOME BIRTH

There is such a variety of options for birthing these days. On one end of the spectrum, there is traditional hospital birth. On the other end, there is unattended home birth. I'm not here to judge how you choose to birth, but I want to be a voice in the crowd cheering for home birth. When I gave birth to my daughter, I had a midwife, a midwife assistant, a doula, and my husband by my side. It was intimate and beautiful.

This is part of the actual journal entry I wrote shortly after having my daughter. I debated sharing this because it's so intimate, but I know there are people who will be empowered by hearing this. I want to be a cheerleader in your corner if you have any hesitation about home birth. You can do it. Your body was made for this.

February 21, 2018:

I was cooking after having cleaned the house the day before. I wanted all the shopping to be done and have some meals ready. As I was baking, I was feeling strong pains in my stomach, but told myself they were Braxton Hicks. People said, "You will know when they are contractions." I was playing with some of the positions we had learned in birthing classes. I found being on my hands and knees to be the most relieving. Throughout the day, the pains happened sporadically.

I told Dakota we should see his parents one more time before the baby came because it was probably going to be a while. His dad was out of town, so it was just his mom. I knew my face was showing the pain if I wasn't squirming to relieve it. I didn't want to give any hints of discomfort to his mom or make her ask any questions. She asked if I had been feeling anything out of the normal. I said no, really thinking it was false labor and not wanting to raise suspicion. On the drive home, the pains got significantly stronger.

We went inside, and I got ready for bed. I asked Dakota to put an app on my phone so I could track contractions, but it turns out I didn't want to track them. I didn't want to see them or know how many or how far apart, so he put the app on his phone and started tracking. He knew when they were coming because I would get on my hands and knees.

I got to the point where I wanted to call Kate (our doula) because she needed a two-hour warning. She asked if I could still talk through contractions, and I said, "I don't know. I haven't been trying to." She asked for statistics, and I told Dakota I didn't want to know them, so he took the phone to the other room and told her. Probably about an hour and a half later, I called again to say I was ready for her to come.

Kate seemed to get there quickly, even though I knew she had a forty-minute drive. She asked when the last time I had eaten was. I ate a little bit of food and went into transition very quickly after that. I had to go poop again and started throwing up at the same time. Dakota was on it. He had the garbage can and was holding my hair back. I started panicking a little and said, "Kate, I need you in here." She came, and I asked her what was happening. She would say things like, "Your body knows what to do. Listen to it," and "You are doing this."

Dakota said it was time to call Terri (our midwife). That was my only indication of how I was progressing. When Terri got there, she started asking some questions about how long it had been since I had eaten and about statistics. I told her I thought I wanted the bath soonish. So they started filling up the tub and getting it ready. Before I got in the tub, Terri wanted to do a cervical check. I told her to tell me before she made contact. I didn't want to be surprised. She checked because I was a first-time mom, and she wanted to make sure it wasn't false labor.

Getting in the pool was almost 100% relief. I only remember having a handful of contractions in the pool. I think I slept a lot when I was in there. I think having them there and them being so comforting and present was what allowed me to relax enough to be able to rest so well. I didn't have to wonder who was going to be there to comfort or give me strength through the next contraction.

The water was slowly losing its power. I told Dakota I wanted to talk to Terri. Later, Terri told me that when he came out to get her, he said, "Your Highness is ready for you." She asked if I was ready to push and if I felt like my body was trying to push. I said no but was willing to try to get *it there. She suggested the toilet. I remember from birthing classes the toilet is muscle memory. They had me sit on the toilet facing the wall so I could rest. Pushing on the toilet felt kind of forced and allowed no rhythm, but I do believe it got the process going.*

I was ready to switch again. I knew I was ready to lay on the bed. I lay on my left side on the edge of the bed. Dakota laid on the bed with me, and he kind of curled against the wall. I am so thankful he didn't get discouraged or back off because I wasn't acknowledging him. He stayed close anyway.

Once I started pushing for real and in rhythm, the midwives stayed in the room, at least one of them at all times. They were checking the heart rate more frequently. Terri told me to try holding my breath for the push. That was probably the most helpful advice through the whole thing. There was a point again where I knew I was getting rest between contractions because I was startled awake by my water breaking. It was a forceful spray, not just a leak, and I heard it pop.

I hit points where the words, "I can't do this," almost came out of my mouth. That was my moment of acceptance. I had to change my thinking. I started saying, "We want you here. We love you. I am ready to have you." She came very quickly after I accepted and started saying that I was ready for her.

I knew it was close, and somehow the actual contractions started hurting less. I was so focused on getting this baby out. Terri was the commentator. She was guiding me on how quickly or slowly to push. I still ripped, but I do think it was helpful to have guidance and even that affirmation of the control I did have.

I yelled during the last handful of pushes. I was on my hands and knees, and they pulled her between my legs right under me.

I just looked at her and repeatedly said, "Oh my goodness." I was in total shock. I picked her up. I leaned against the wall and held her.

I interviewed at least five midwives before I found mine. I knew what I wanted my home birth to look like, and I wasn't willing to settle for "good enough." That can be the difference between a good experience and a bad one. If you know what it is you want, do your research, ask around, and interview lots.

Being pregnant and giving birth is one of the times everyone thinks they have permission to speak into your life. I want to be a voice and inspiration that says you have a choice. You don't have to give birth any certain way or the way society says. God designed our bodies to do this, and if we let our bodies do their job, they know what to do. I am thankful for the people who came alongside me and encouraged me in my choice.

ACTION:

1. Are you making your health a priority? Why or why not?

2. What is one way you can respect your body more? What is it communicating to you?

3. Are there any changes you've been wanting to make but haven't yet? What is stopping you from making those changes?

4. What does the best version of yourself look like? Visualize the inside and outside of yourself. How do they go together?

10

MAKING AN INTENTIONAL SCHEDULE

Over the years, I have gone through a cycle more times than I would like to admit. I will find habits and routines that keep me balanced. I'll build up my capacity physically, mentally, and spiritually, and when I am feeling good, I'll let the habits and behaviors that helped me feel good in the first place slide. The same is true when it comes to my daughter's schedule. She will be thriving, so I will let our routine slip until it is nonexistent. I let myself forget that the reason she is doing so well is because of the structure.

When I am doing well, feeling good, and in a healthy brain space, I need to keep doing the things that got me there. Creating a routine and being purposeful about the way I spend my days helps ensure I am healthy physically, mentally, and spiritually.

I want to give you a template for a daily routine. Sometimes, not knowing where to start hinders us from starting at all. This is what works for our little family and our natural rhythms in this season. Adjust it for what works for your family. If you try this and hate it, you'll still have a better sense of what you are looking for.

6:00 a.m.–7:00 a.m.	Mommy time
7:00 a.m.–7:30 a.m.	Read with Kennedy
7:30 a.m.–7:45 a.m.	Get ready for the day
7:45 a.m.–8:15 a.m.	Breakfast
8:15 a.m.–8:45 a.m.	Learning/intentional playtime

8:45 a.m.–9:00 a.m.	Small chores
9:00 a.m.–10:00 a.m.	Outdoor time
10:00 a.m.–10:15 a.m.	Snack
10:15 a.m.–12:00 p.m.	Project or outing
12:00 p.m.–1:00 p.m.	Lunch and prep for Kennedy's nap
1:00 p.m.–3:00 p.m.	Naptime
3:00 p.m.–4:30 p.m.	Project, park, or less-structured play
4:30 p.m.–5:30 p.m.	Dinner prep
5:30 p.m.–6:00 p.m.	Dinner
6:00 p.m.–6:30 p.m.	Undivided playtime with Daddy/clean the kitchen
6:30 p.m.–6:40 p.m.	Tidy up house
6:40 p.m.–7:00 p.m.	Shower/prep for bed
7:00 p.m.–9:00 p.m.	Mom's activity time
9:00 p.m.–10:00 p.m.	Read in bed

MOMMY TIME

One of the things that helps me have a strong body and mind is to have a few minutes to myself in the morning. I have gone through seasons where I wanted to sleep until the very last second before my daughter woke up. What I've learned about myself as a mom is I want to be available for her first thing when she wakes up. I want those first wake-up snuggles. In order to do that fully, I need to set aside time for myself first.

The first thing I do when I roll out of bed is work out. If I don't work out first thing, it usually doesn't happen.

I took a mama and baby yoga class once, and the instructor said if all you do is child's pose for ten minutes, you have succeeded. She said that once you are in the pose, it will flow from there. I have that in my mind on days I don't particularly feel like stretching. I tell myself all I have to do is child's pose. Once I'm there, it does flow. My body begins to ask for what it needs, and it is so easy to stretch for ten minutes.

Oftentimes, it is needing to make the decision to start that holds us back. We tell ourselves, "I don't know what stretches I will do," "I don't know enough stretches for ten minutes," or "I only know basic stretches." Put all excuses out of the way. Embrace the idea that all you have to do is child's pose. Maybe that's all you do. Once it is a routine, you can expand from there.

Next, I have time for reading and prayer. I want to be in the presence of God first thing in the morning and invite Him into my day. I like reading in the morning because it puts the words of God into my mind. You don't have to memorize the verses for them to reframe your thinking. It's wild how much I enjoy reading my Bible when I haven't always in the past. I have struggled with being legalistic, so reading the Bible used to be like reading a list of rules. Now when I read, I can't wait to see what happens next and what God is saying to me.

I also start my day with affirmations. I put sticky notes all over my bathroom mirror. I have an automatic toothbrush that goes for two minutes, so I put those two minutes to work and read my notes while brushing my teeth. Now, if I finish brushing my teeth and I haven't read my affirmations, it feels like something is missing. In a house we used to rent, there was a bathroom where the toilet faced the mirror. So, we read affirmations while going potty. (This might be TMI. Sorry, not sorry.) Look out for the spaces of time you can use, like when you might otherwise be scrolling through your phone. What are the times you are looking to fill? Fill them with affirmations.

Wrapping up my quiet time can go one of a few ways: Sometimes I am inspired to journal. Sometimes I will pick up my just-for-me book. A lot of times, Kennedy is just waking up. If she is about to wake up, I won't start a new activity. I know I am much more patient with her if I'm not in the middle of something when she crawls out of bed.

I am intentional about not picking up my phone during this morning mommy time. Maybe you can relate to the experience of getting up, immediately checking your phone, and being emotionally charged by what appears. I want to protect this time. This small object can have such a sway in my emotions.

When I'm deciding how I want to spend my mornings, the image of a balance beam comes to mind. Let's say when you wake up, you start with a balance beam that's three inches wide, but you can take steps to add to that width. You get a cup of coffee or tea, and your balance beam widens by two inches. You stretch, and you add two more. You read, journal, or meditate, and again you add two inches. Now, when you open the door and walk out into the world, you are much less likely to lose your balance. You've created a solid path to steady your steps. Your balance beam resets each morning, so you have to keep doing the things that keep you on a grounded, steady path.

How you spend your mornings can determine the course of your day.

READ WITH KENNEDY

This is an idea I have heard from multiple moms: if you give your kids undivided attention at the beginning of the day, they usually behave better throughout the day. Why does it work? I think it's because you're filling up their "love tank." This time is about so much more than reading. I am showing my daughter I will make time for her every day.

When we are intentionally present with our little ones, it sets the tone for the entire day. It puts into focus what's important. It not only helps us slow down at that moment but helps us be more in tune all day.

GET READY FOR THE DAY

Some people say you should get dressed before eating breakfast. I agree. Wearing pajamas tells your brain it's time to go to sleep. Getting ready for your day is a good way to kick-start your brain. Even if you aren't 100% sure of what the day holds, you'll be ready for whatever it is. You'll be ready to go on an outing, answer the front door, or have a spontaneous playdate. If you answer the door feeling frumpy, it negatively impacts your mind. Getting ready for your day, even if you don't happen to answer the front door, positively impacts your mind. It's okay to feel cute when no one else sees you. It makes a difference how you feel about yourself, even when you're in your own house.

BREAKFAST

Being intentional and starting your day off right with healthy food will curb and even eliminate your craving for unhealthy foods later in the day. Sometimes, we think the only thing that will taste good is something that's bad for us when really, we can make delicious, good-for-us food and be pleasantly surprised that it fills the craving. It is better for our mental and physical health. At the time, it might not feel like vegetables can compare to sugar, but in the end, it's about so much more than the flavor. Not only did I eat good food, but I feel proud of my choices. My brain feels better for days afterward. I am reinforcing that I am strong.

LEARNING/INTENTIONAL PLAYTIME

Earlier in this book, I told you about my struggle to stay present while playing with my daughter. This is one of the things in my life I have had to work the hardest on and having structure around it has been so helpful. In the beginning, I found that setting a physical timer was a big help. It released me from checking the clock and helped me stay engaged from beginning to end. I stopped checking out early because we were nearly done with our playtime. I stopped being frantic and flustered about how much time was left. It eliminated variables and allowed me to be present.

SMALL CHORES

This is a time for those little chores that are going to nag you all day if you don't just do them. Use this time to start the laundry, take that box to the car, put the letter in the mail, throw the recycling in the blue bin, whatever it is that needs to be done today.

OUTDOOR TIME

This is the part of our day where we do all our outdoor chores. We water the plants, feed the animals, and complete any pressing next steps in the garden. Even if you don't have any outdoor chores you need to complete, I would still recommend spending this time outdoors. Go to a park or on a walk. Everyone should have at least thirty minutes of fresh air a day. Having it in the schedule raises your commitment. Even if you look out your window and the weather is encouraging you to stay in, I still challenge you to go out anyway. I had a teacher at the nature school I attended who would say, "There is no bad weather, only bad clothing." I love this!

Embrace all the seasons and weather. Make time in your day to connect with the earth and the elements.

I don't want to leave this subject without adding that we are electromagnetic beings. We are energy. There are so many studies that show the health benefits of being in nature and grounding or earthing. This is simply removing barriers between you and the earth. Take off your shoes or lay in the grass.

Because there is no such thing as bad weather, my daughter and I play in whatever the weather brings. When there were forest fires this summer, and the air was thick with smoke, she prayed for rain. When the rain came, she danced around and squealed with excitement, proclaiming God had answered her prayers.

Don't let your day slip by without outdoor time. However you spend it—exercising, gardening, shoveling snow, raking leaves, laying in the grass, singing with the birds—let it fill you. After all, we were perfectly designed to live in nature.

SNACK

Having planned food times has been a powerful experience for me. Because there was scarcity in my childhood, I always wanted my children to have access to food when they were hungry. I was so driven to make sure her story wasn't the same as mine, I let my daughter have food all day long. I am finding there is a healthy way to put boundaries around food. Children feel more secure with boundaries. They are looking for us to set limits lovingly.

Sometimes, I have to fight myself to keep these boundaries, and it is hard. My emotions will tell me that the most loving thing I can do is to give my daughter what I needed as a child. When I do this, I am parenting out of my pain. I want to parent out of wholeness.

PROJECT OR OUTING

I like to lay out my calendar by having a theme for the week. I'll look at the month and to-do list to decide the theme and then write it to the side of each week. Maybe the theme is getting seeds in the ground. In that week's to-do list, I'll write the smaller tasks that go along with this main goal.

I struggle with overbooking. I pack so much into the day that I end up missing out on my life. I miss out on time with my family and on resting. By keeping my projects contained to a specific time, I am more realistic about what I can get done in a day, and I stop when the time is done.

We also have regular weekly outings. This helps give us rhythm and things to look forward to. I do better when I know we have an outing coming up, even if it is days away. Even though I could leave the house any day of the week, it helps me to have a set plan.

LUNCH AND PREP FOR KENNEDY'S NAP

I sometimes find it difficult to set aside this time. I tell myself it won't take that long to make lunch or get Kennedy ready for her nap or a million other excuses to shorten this time. The problem is I inevitably end up rushing and getting frustrated. I'll end up getting Kennedy down late for her nap and messing up the afternoon schedule. Then, later in the day, she won't be ready for bed on time. It usually takes two or three days to get back on track when we adjust a sleeping period.

Our default is to get frustrated at our children when they are having trouble behaving or have negative attitudes. This was a huge reminder for me that, as parents, it is our job and responsibility to set them up for success. If I change the schedule I know sets Kennedy up for success, then I have to take responsibility for the poor behavior.

NAPTIME

There was a time when I thought Kennedy was growing out of naps. It turned out to be the lack of a schedule that made it difficult for her to rest. When I put the schedule back into place, she started napping regularly and predictably. A naptime or quiet time can solve a lot of problems. Even if your kids don't nap, it is still good for them to have a time of rest. Quiet time is good for parents too.

PROJECT, PARK, OR LESS-STRUCTURED PLAY

This is another time of day when if there are small chores that need to get done, you can bust them out. If it's a day where you just need to snuggle with your child, play a game, or do some crafts, that is great too. Maybe you have some more outside time or independent play. You can use this time for whatever fits best that day.

DINNER PREP

This is probably my weakest area. Sometimes (a lot of times), the less structured part of our day will spill over into this time. If I have a meal plan, I am great at getting in the kitchen and making it happen. If I don't have a plan, it is often Dakota who cooks because he is the creative cook. He makes the most delicious meals out of whatever we have on hand.

DINNER

I am a firm believer in having dinner at the table with no electronics. It benefits our kids to have dinner as a family. It is a simple way to spend intentional time together. I love it when our toddler states very clearly that there are no phones allowed at the table. It is funny and cute to see her say this, but it also makes me proud. I love seeing her have a high standard for our meals together. In every aspect of the way we raise our kids, we are teaching them what to expect and what standards to keep.

UNDIVIDED PLAYTIME WITH DADDY/CLEAN THE KITCHEN

I feel blessed that I don't work a traditional job and can stay home and spend my days with my daughter. It makes me sad to think about how few hours a day my husband gets to spend with her. I want to make the most of the time they do have together. I have come to enjoy the few minutes I spend cleaning the kitchen alone while they play one-on-one. I love hearing them giggle. They need uninterrupted time to spend together.

TIDY UP HOUSE

We are calmer and more relaxed when we have picked up spaces. One practice that works for us is to have a ten-to-fifteen-minute pickup session every night. It's amazing the transformation that can take place in ten minutes. It's important that everything in your house has a home. Then, it won't be a matter of deciding where things go; it will be a matter of putting things where they go. It's also important that everyone in your house knows where things go. That way, everyone can pitch in.

It is so nice to wake up to a tidy house and just breathe.

SHOWER/PREP FOR BED

Early on after becoming parents, I handed over Kennedy's hygiene routine to Dakota. As moms, it can be hard to give up the tasks we perceive as being "our job." Or maybe we just feel like we can do it better. It is okay to let our men figure it out. It might feel awkward, and it may be hard not to step in and take over, but that can end up making our partners feel inadequate. They are as much a parent as we are, and it is so beneficial for them to be engaged in this way. Encourage them and let them do it on their own.

MOM'S ACTIVITY TIME

If I don't have a plan for my evening once Kennedy is in bed, I will get nothing done. I get caught in the trap of thinking when the baby is down, the night is over. This isn't all bad. There should be nights of rest. Also, I recognize how much time I lose to TV or social media if there isn't a plan. In my calendar, I have three chunks in my day. At the top of each day, I write a main goal for the three different parts of my day. Right now this is so beautifully divided by my child's sleep schedule. We have morning, after nap, and after she goes to bed. This is a rough draft of my goals to get your ideas flowing:

> Monday: Garbage walk, chores, community group
> Tuesday: Community brunch, counseling, Bible study
> Wednesday: Date day with Kennedy, meal plan, read parenting
> book with Dakota

Thursday: Grocery shop, food prep, clean the house
Friday: Self-care, fun project/craft, date night
Saturday: Family and project day
Sunday: Sabbath/Rest

This might change every month. Maybe there are certain things you do once a month or every other week. Maybe you schedule extra free time during some weeks. This system helps me prioritize my main goals and commitments.

I also like this system because, in the past, I'd book things back-to-back, not caring if my days were booked as long as my activities didn't overlap. Something I am learning is to book less for myself. I don't want to live my life rushed. Now I plan one main activity for each chunk of my day and no more. I choose to slow down and not say yes to something just because I can fit it in. Just because it can fit into a time slot doesn't mean it is healthy for me emotionally or physically.

I used to never consider saying no to an activity if my schedule was open. If there wasn't something interfering, I would say yes. If someone asked, I would give up any "me time" because I didn't consider that time booked. I'd justify this by reasoning I could take "me time" anytime. Now, I book time for myself first. I have to take care of myself first if I want to help others. I can't help them at the expense of myself.

READ IN BED

This is probably one of the most relaxing things I do for myself, and I love finishing my day this way. I've made it a practice to crawl into bed, read, and let my body settle down naturally. I may fall asleep in ten minutes, or I may read for an hour. Reading is something that makes me feel like I poured into myself. It is a great way to be gentle with and value myself. It helps me go to sleep relaxed and refreshed.

Even though I'm not a night person, it can be hard for me to go to bed on time. I know myself well enough to know my schedule works so much better when I do go to bed early. I am happier, more patient, and more content when I stick to the plan and give my body what it needs. Reading in bed is one of the ways I encourage myself to fall asleep when I need to.

DOING WHAT MAKES YOU
HAPPY IN ALL SEASONS

I live in the Pacific Northwest, and we get short days in the wintertime. So many people get down in the wintertime, and when the sun comes back, they come back to life. It is a common pattern that feeds into the high highs and low lows I already experience.

If there's something that makes you happy in the summer, find a way to do it in the winter too. I love going on walks, so when there is snow on the ground, I can feel a little cooped up. Those walks and the endorphins they give me are so important to my mental health. If I can't walk outside, I need to find another way to exercise. It starts with giving up the little things when the seasons change, and soon we are giving up many little rhythms that make us happy. Be diligent and don't let this happen.

A lot of times your activities will have to change, yes, but replace them with something you will look forward to equally. Come winter, our garden will fade, and the bees will be in for the season, but I will be saving the beeswax all summer for a project I can do in the fall or winter. I will have sewing projects and books to study.

Make plans that give purpose and direction to every month of the year. Fill your schedule with activities that will bring you joy.

> January: Make a seed-starting calendar and organize the seeds by when they need to be planted.
> February: Plan Kennedy and Dakota's birthday party.
> March: Put your starts in the greenhouse.
> April: Prep the garden.
> May: Plant the garden.
> June: Plan playdates and summer fun.
> July: Plant the fall crop and clean/organize the basement.
> August: Plan and organize Kennedy's school.
> September: Clean up the garden and add organic material.
> October: Update, clean out, and add new recipes to my cookbook.
> November: Make Christmas gifts (I love making gifts. I usually make a lot of one thing I think everyone should have. For example, last year it was reusable car garbage bags.) and Christmas cards.
> December: Make this year's scrapbook.

ACTION:

1. What are the habits that make you feel physically, mentally, and spiritually healthy? Add these things to your schedule.

2. Try making your own schedule. Follow it for a week and adjust if necessary.

3. If there are activities you enjoy in summer that you can't enjoy in winter, what are some of the ways you can replace those summer activities?

4. Make a list of activities you can look forward to for each month of the year.

11

BRINGING ONLY POSITIVITY INTO YOUR SPACE

In elementary school, my class was given the assignment to not watch TV for one week. I was so excited. Even from a young age, I felt wary of TV. My mom was on board and willing to support me in my assignment. I was devastated when I realized she didn't consider movies to be the same as TV, and we had movies playing that week. The experience impacted me profoundly. I longed for a break from TV and movies, even as a kid. I still feel that as an adult.

We do not own a television. For years, we kept the TV in an armoire or a spare room. Eventually, we booted it completely. Our culture allows TV, media, and advertisements to leak into our brains subconsciously. I don't even want to know how many ads we take in daily. Everywhere we turn, our world is bombarding us with messages, and those messages have an agenda. I am not okay with handing over my mental real estate to a presence that has no interest in me.

This may be surprising to hear since earlier in this book, I told you about the important lessons I have found in movies and TV shows. It's when approaching media with purpose and making it the exception, not the rule, that you find the messages that will serve you. You have control over the messages in your space.

Take some time to write down your answers to these questions:

1. What is TV giving you? What is it taking?
2. Look back at your first answer. Circle the positive things. Do the positives outweigh the negatives?
3. If you weren't watching TV, what would you replace that time with? Even if you don't watch that much TV now, how can you replace that time with activities that will fill you up?
4. What are three to five things that you find yourself saying, "I'll do that when I have time"? Challenge yourself to do one of these activities in place of watching TV.

I'd like to challenge you to take a week-long break from TV. When I say TV, I mean movies too. Each day of that week, take notice of how you feel. After a week, look back and consider if your time was more productive, less distracted, more planned, more intentional, more social, more physical, or more creative. What was it more of, and what was it less of?

Guys, I know some of you are saying, "This activity isn't for me. I don't watch that much TV." I challenge you to try anyway.

PHONE-OFF DAY

I started implementing phone-off days during one of the busiest seasons of my life. I was managing a bookstore, cleaning people's homes, being a mommy, and taking care of the house while my husband worked out of town four to five days a week. I needed one day that nobody needed anything from me. I didn't want to feel obligated to respond to anyone.

When I exchange numbers with someone, I warn them I'm not a committed texter. My best friends know if I haven't responded to a text in three days and it's urgent, they should call. I generally have no less than fifteen unopened texts at any given time. When I do open them and respond to everyone, they all message back, and I'm right back where I started. So, I just turn my phone off, and it relieves some of the tension. My husband is great at setting aside issues he doesn't have energy for that day. He says, "That's a problem for tomorrow's Dakota." I have adopted this, and sometimes it is just the freedom I need to let "tomorrow's Amie" take care of it.

When I'm inside my home, it rejuvenates me to let my brain rest from the nagging of the world. Home is supposed to be the place we rest and prepare to take on the world. When we take down that barrier and allow constant intrusions, we have no safe space. I don't have control over what others say and do, but I do have control over what I allow in my space.

Another reason I do a phone off-day is to give perspective to the days I have it on. When your phone is off, notice how many times a day you think about grabbing it or going to look for it. The artist Eric Pickersgill did a photo series that shows what we look like in day-to-day life, but he removed the devices from the photos. The one that stuck out to me the most was the one where a husband and wife are lying in bed back-to-back, looking at their cupped hands.[32]

How does having our phones off change our interactions with our family? How many times a day do we tell our kids, "Hang on just a minute," while we are doing something on our phones? How many of our conversations with our spouses are spent looking at a screen instead of making eye contact?

Having a phone-off day is a valuable exercise. Maybe your phone is a comfort to you. Maybe it's a pacifier, a distraction, a coping mechanism, a confidence-booster, etc. Who are you without it, and how are you different? Electronics have taken a piece of our human connection with each other and with ourselves.

You have power. You have control. Fight for your well-being.

BOOKS

I have heard many people say, "I wish I had more time to read." When you are considering whether to do a phone-off day or reduce the amount of TV you watch, remember that more time to read is one of the benefits you get. It is a way to add more value to your life intentionally.

I love books. There are so many amazing resources and so much access to knowledge. Audiobooks have made it easier than ever, whether you listen to them while doing chores, exercising, or driving. I had a group of friends that called audiobooks "car university." They estimated that in a

---

[32] Eric Pickersgill, *Ange and Me,* 2014, Removed. https://www.ericpickersgill.com/removed.

year, you spend close to the same number of hours in your car as it takes to get a degree.

Years ago, I was challenged to read fifteen minutes a day, and it has been one of my daily goals ever since. There are so many good books out there. For me, it is hard to choose what to read next because I have such a long to-be-read list. I think that list grows faster than I read through it, but it is worth it. If you have a book list, fantastic! If you don't, I want to give you a boost by suggesting ways to create your own.

When I'm talking to someone and they mention a book, I always make at least a mental note. I have some friends whose reading interests align with mine, and I will read any book they recommend. I have some friends who don't like the same types of books as I do, and that's okay. I just try to identify which friends share my reading tastes. Then I keep a mental note of their referrals.

If I am reading a book I really like, I will note the books the author references. I always note those books in a special place so I remember them. There are so many good books, so I have to be selective about what makes it onto my to-be-read list. There are some books I like, but not enough to add the references to my list. If a book has come up for me at least three times, whether in a conversation or in a reference, that tells me it is one I should look into.

Another way to decide if you want to read a book is to look at who the forward is written by. When I was a new reader, the forwards meant nothing to me because I wasn't familiar with very many authors. Now, I find them invaluable. I have read some great books I never would have taken a second look at if I hadn't recognized the person who wrote the forward.

Sometimes, you may like an author, but you won't like the books they endorse. I even find sometimes that the authors they are supporting are distasteful. When you're getting to know an author, look into what type of messages they promote. They may no longer be an author you want to follow.

You can learn a lot about an author by listening to their podcasts. It can be a podcast they are the host of or an episode where they make a guest appearance. It is a great way to get a feel for an author and what they are passionate about. Even if their podcast focuses more on hosting or interviewing other people, you will learn a lot about them. You can learn a lot about someone by the way they interact with other people.

At the end of this book, I have created a list of some of my favorite titles. This list can be a possible jumping-off point for you, but don't fill up your Amazon cart with every book on the list and spend a thousand dollars. Maybe get one. While you are reading that book, check your local thrift store or garage sales for other titles on your list. By the time you are done with the first one, you might have one or two more. This is how I've built a lot of my collection. I have an ongoing list of the books I'm looking out for, and when I find them for a good deal, I get them.

There are so many good books in the world. On the other hand, I have had to learn to give myself permission to leave a book incomplete. A book can hurt your spirit more than heal it. I used to have a really hard time not finishing a book. I wanted to be able to put it on my bookshelf with my other finished books. If it isn't the right season for a book or never will be, let it go. If it isn't life-giving, let it go. Disclaimer: life-giving doesn't mean not challenging.

I have expanded my skillset and knowledge so much through reading. I am learning from people who are living in their strengths and taking the time to make their ideas accessible to all. Take advantage of the resources surrounding you. If I'm reluctant to spend money on a book, I ask myself, "Will I be X amount of dollars smarter?" I see it as paying for knowledge, not an item. I am investing in the person I want to be, and that is so worth the money. Remember, you are buying gold.

MY GOLD: FINISHED BOOK QUOTES

I have come to think of the information that impacts me the most as my gold. There is a lot of gold out there. We all have different interests and would potentially view different types of knowledge as gold.

This is one of my all-time favorite practices. It is my gold for you. I have a notebook that is a collection of my gold. Every time I finish reading or listening to a book, I log it in my notebook. I write the title, the author, and the date I finished it. Then I write down the quotes I highlighted in the book.

You know the question, "What would you grab if your house was on fire and you could only take one thing?" Assuming my family is safe, the first thing that comes to mind is my notebook. I look back and am so thankful I started this a long time ago. At the time, I didn't realize what it would turn into. Now, I am even more grateful that I have it.

If I open my notebook and start reading the quotes, it is suddenly like I am reading a whole new book. I sometimes get more from my page of highlights than from a whole book. The quotes are ones I've handpicked and are specifically what I need. Writing the quotes down also engages a different part of your brain and helps commit them to memory.

I so value the reflection I do when I write these quotes down. Sometimes I'll finish a book and think, "Meh, it wasn't my favorite." The book sits on the shelf, waiting for me to transfer the quotes to my notebook. Sometimes it will take months for me to pick it up again. Finally, I do because I'm tired of not having the task complete. When I read through the quotes, they hit me in a way they didn't before. Something about the break makes them more powerful. I end up wondering why the book isn't one of my favorites. Whatever the reason, I am thankful for the system that makes me circle back.

My gold book is also a great resource when I'm trying to remember where I learned something. Often, I'll only remember part of a quote and want to go back and refresh. I also turn to it when I am writing encouraging notes. It makes it so easy to find motivational quotes and source them quickly. When I finish a book, I have lots of ideas and connections firing in my brain, and I like having this resource to keep track of where everything came from. I am better at recommending books because of it as well.

This personalized book tells so much about me without using any of my own words. You can see the progression of my journey, my interests, my longings, and my challenges. It is a map of my life.

This book of quotes is kind of like scrapbooking. I see it as collecting the pieces and putting them together in a way that makes my own art. It is cutting and gluing all the pieces that tell my story in words I didn't have before. I can discover myself in other people's words.

FILL YOUR SPACE WITH AFFIRMATION

Back in 2020, when we chose to stay in our current house and start our farm here, we were just one day away from listing the house. We had been preparing to move for months, and we had started packing everything away. I remember looking around the emptying house and thinking it was beautiful, but it was starting to feel lifeless.

We experienced the feeling of having a clear, depersonalized house. I had thought it would be nice to live in a house that was put together and picture-perfect. I was surprised to find it was draining.

Do you know that feeling when you walk into a really cute boutique, and you ogle at everything on the shelves? You just can't get over the feel, the colors, or the smell. It captures you, and you can't get over how you feel standing there. This is how your home should feel when you open the front door. I can see some eyes rolling right now, but I'm here to tell you it is attainable. And oh, how much I want to help you. If I could jump through the pages and work on your house with you for a week, I would. It is so important for your mind, mood, energy level, motivation, creativity, and so much more to have a space you love.

Is there a color that makes you feel cozy and happy? Try painting an accent wall with that color. Is there a smell that makes you feel safe or calm? Find the things that evoke some reaction in you and recreate them in your own way. Try walking through a vendor mall. You can see many people's styles all in one place and find what stands out to you.

My dad taught me to hang pictures to remind me of the good times. In my own home, I like to make sure those pictures are rotating. I don't like getting used to them being there. Once I get used to them, I stop noticing them. My favorite decoration is a picture frame filled with photos from my husband and I's honeymoon. Surrounding it are pictures of us on each of our anniversaries.

Putting affirmations in your space is a way to lift your spirits. Philippians 4:8 says, "Fix your thoughts on what is true, and honorable, and right, and pure, and lovely, and admirable. Think about things that are excellent and worthy of praise."[33] My bathroom mirror is covered with sticky notes with positive thoughts written on them. Whiteboard markers erase off of mirrors, so the mirror itself has affirmations too. On the window of our back door, the door that leads out to the garden, I wrote a blessing from Deuteronomy 33 about the abundance of the land. I have

---

[33] Philippians 4:8 (New Living Translation).
<u>Conclusion</u>

prayer cards with verses written in cute colors and letters. I laminated some and have them tucked behind the light switch covers. Kennedy and I pained some rocks that we will write promises on and put around our garden. There are endless ways to incorporate positive thoughts and promises around your home.

Get creative. Claim your home. You will reflect how your space feels, and your space will reflect how you feel.

WHAT STILL SERVES YOU?

On the flip side, it is just as important to remove things from your home that affect you negatively. Our things can weigh on us. It is important to evaluate often if what you have is still your favorite.

One of the things I tell the clients I clean for is, "If it *was* your favorite, it never will be again, so let it go." I learned this for myself after going through many moves. I would hold on to something just because it had once been my favorite, maybe even years ago. I would move these things with us, and when we went to move again, I would find myself repeating the same pattern.

It's okay to let these things go. Just because it was your favorite doesn't mean you have to hold onto it forever. You can actually feel good about getting rid of it because you have made good use of that thing. Multiple times, I have seen the same look of, "But it was my favorite" on clients' faces. Eventually, they would put it in the get-rid-of box. We grow out of our favorites. It feels better to let them go rather than hang on to them, hoping they will be our favorite again.

As much as I am against wasting, it is necessary to flip my mindset when I am organizing. Get a pack of your favorite pens and get rid of the drawer full of them. Same with hair ties. Don't have a whole pack strewn about. Have one hair tie until you wear it out. Keep track of it and put it away because you can't get another one until this one stretches out or breaks. Have one item that is your favorite instead of multiple you like. Having less clutter will impact how you feel.

If you are trying to make a lifestyle change, such as living more sustainably, get rid of anything that goes against the change you want to make. If you know you don't want plastic in your house anymore, get rid of it. Make a list of what you want to replace. This can be hard for me when I'm worried about being wasteful. I'll hold onto a box of cotton swabs even when I know I want to get reusable ones. Get rid of it. It is affecting you. Let go of the life you don't want to live and replace it with the life you do want to live. There is tension in you when these things are half done. It might feel hard to make the decision and take the donation box out the front door, but I promise you it will feel so much better when it is dropped off.

Schedule the time to do a deep clean. Pull everything out and decide if it is still having a positive impact on your life. This is why I didn't mind moving so much for years. Every year, we'd pack everything we had into boxes and relocate. Most people offered their sympathies, but I enjoyed it. When you have to put something in a box and move it, it helps you decide if you really want it.

One of the reasons I like helping people clean and organize is because it is such an intimidating task for so many people. It feels too big. Some people start thinking it won't be that bad, and about three-quarters of the way through, they want to light the house on fire. It is a big undertaking, so start with little steps. Start in just one room and take everything out. Take things off of shelves, out of closets and drawers, out from underneath the bed, and off the door. Even take the pictures off the walls. This is how anyone can transform their home.

I will break down my tips for organizing and cleaning in the next section. For now, I want to emphasize how much your space affects your mental health. You need to prioritize how it makes you feel. I know it's hard to get the energy and motivation, but it will pay you back exponentially in your daily life. It will pay you back far more than it will cost you.

ACTION:

1. Try doing a phone-off day one day a week for a month. Write down your observations. How did your mental health change? How did your relationships change?

2. Start a book list. What are some books you've heard about a few times that have piqued your interest?

3. The next time you read a book, highlight or write down your favorite quotes. Keep your gold in a safe and accessible place.

4. Schedule a day to go out, be intentional, and take notes. Take in the smells, colors, and styles you see. Notice what you are drawn to and begin to transform your home.

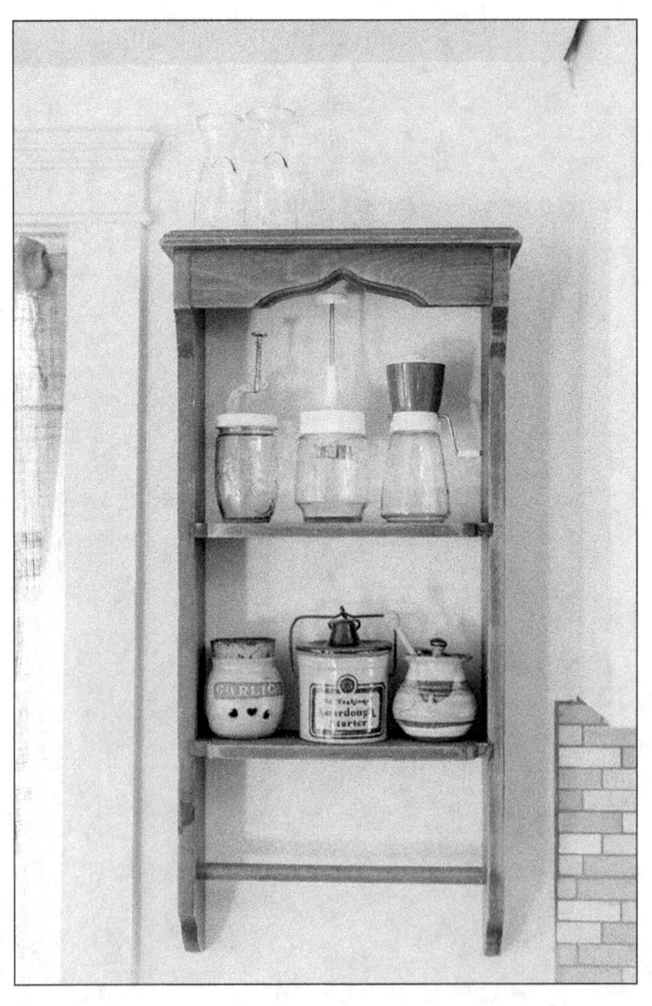
GARLIC
Sourdough
Starter

PART 4

CREATING SYSTEMS FOR YOUR HOME AND LIFE

12

MAKING HEALTHY CHOICES EASY

In Part 3, we started talking about the importance of what you eat and its connection to your mental health. The reality is that making lasting and meaningful changes to your diet can be hard. It takes time and accountability.

No matter what your goals are or how you want to change your diet, I'd encourage you to get a tool kit. Hope isn't going to get you very far. You need to have a plan. Build a support system of people who can cheer you on and keep you accountable. Make a meal plan, get a food diary, or find whatever resources will make you feel the most supported.

The Paleo lifestyle has given me confidence and pride in how I eat. Find the food that gives you confidence and pride. My naturopathic doctor talks a lot about the connection between our brains and our guts. When I listen to my body, feed it well, and honor it when it is full, I feel better about food in general. This creates a cycle of wanting to eat healthier food and stop eating when I'm full. It is making new neural pathways that associate portion control and vegetables with positive feelings.

This path to change can be an uphill climb, so it's important to set yourself up for success. Let's dive into some practical tools and ideas for a more attainable, positive food journey.

HAVE SYSTEMS IN PLACE

In my experience, people tend to make poor eating choices when they don't have systems of organization for their food. You know when someone walks into a room and asks where everybody is, but they are only looking for one or two people? Food can be that way. If you don't have your favorite go-to snack or meal, you feel like you have no options. You have a few little things that make it feel like you have a variety of choices, and if you don't have those, your cupboard might as well be empty.

It is key to recognize what these foods are for you. For me, it is having leftovers, walnuts or almonds, and bananas or apples. When you know what foods help you feel comfortable and like you're living in abundance, you'll make better choices for your health.

This relates back to the connection between our brain and gut. When my mind switches into scarcity mode, I start overeating. This is true even if I have a pantry full of food. It is worth going to the store and spending ten to twenty dollars to buy the few things that keep my mind in a good place. I don't need to go on a two-hundred-dollar shopping spree; I just need a few things. Notice when you're asking yourself, "Where is all the food?" What is it you are really looking for?

This is also an opportunity to start making small shifts in your diet. For example, if your go-to snack is potato chips, try kale or apple chips. Find healthy replacements for those go-to snacks. Here are some healthy alternatives you can try:

- Carrots or celery with nut butter
- Apples or peaches with nut butter
- Bananas with walnuts
- Almonds, walnuts, cashews, or peanuts
- Hard-boiled eggs
- Olives
- Pumpkin seeds
- Homemade trail mix
- Homemade granola (for a special treat to keep as a safety net)
- Quinoa with seeds and nuts
- Plant milk topped with fruit, quinoa, seeds, and nuts

Once you have a few go-to options that align with your lifestyle, let's talk about leaving the house. Always bring a snack with you. When I first switched to a gluten-free diet, I often felt left out. I would compromise and eat something because I was feeling insecure, not because I was hungry. If I have my own snacks, I feel empowered to only eat when I am hungry. Just knowing it's there makes me feel more secure. I can go past the surface-level question of, "What will I eat?" to ask, "Am I even hungry?"

I also keep backup snacks in my outing backpack. If for some reason I don't have the backpack, I have more snacks in the car. I don't want to compromise on food because I didn't plan well. I keep systems in place to help me when I am forgetful.

Also, make food easy and accessible at home. This is why I love our open-concept kitchen cupboards. I store food in glass containers for two reasons: One, I don't want to have plastic in our home. Two, it makes great décor. With how much dehydrating we do, we just keep ongoing snack jars. They work beautifully for bulk foods as well. I just pour the bulk food into their jars. Having healthy options available and accessible makes it easier to make good choices. When you feel good about the choices you're making, you continue to make good choices.

Eating healthy is about mental health as much as gut health. Usually, when someone is struggling with food, the roots of why are way deeper. Having healthy, accessible options can make this easier and more attainable. You aren't simply retraining your taste buds. You are breaking down old habits and mindsets and fighting for a better version of yourself. Fighting for your physical health is a holistic process. You can't just change your actions. You have to change your beliefs.

Give yourself as many advantages as possible. If you knew you were going for a fifty-mile hike, you would pick all your gear methodically (at least I hope you would). You would get the most efficient and effective tools and would leave behind the things that would weigh you down. You would probably have a list and do a lot of prepping.

It is your responsibility to get the tools you need. Don't leave any excuses for you to fail. Plan for success. Jump all in.

THE EAT-ME-FIRST BIN

I have a bin labeled "Eat Me First," and it is probably one of the best inventions my fridge has ever come up with. Before I go grocery shopping, I put any remaining produce into this bin. This is so when the new food gets home and washed up, there is no guessing what needs to be used first. It helps my new food last longer because if something does start to go bad, it isn't sitting next to the new stuff.

I used to have this mental block about throwing food away. I'd only throw it away if there was something growing on it. I would keep food I'd already decided I wasn't going to eat. It was bad. Routines help create good habits. Having a regular shopping schedule helps me remember to clean the fridge out before I put new stuff in. The Eat-Me-First bin gives food one last chance before it gets composted or fed to the chickens. It also prevents me from letting food sit in the fridge forever.

Having this bin has significantly decreased our food waste. I am constantly evaluating what needs to be used. It's a reminder to check and see if there is anything we can add to our meal or an item we can base a meal around. It keeps things localized, so nothing slips through the cracks.

NEW COOKBOOKS

When I get a new cookbook, I comb through it and tag the recipes I think I could manage immediately. These are recipes where I recognize most of the ingredients and would be comfortable implementing that meal next week. Even if the recipe stretches me a little bit and has one or two things I don't know how to do, it doesn't feel totally daunting. I tag those recipes with a sticky note at the top of the page.

Next, I tag the recipes I want to try but would take significantly more commitment. I tag those on the side of the page. Depending on how ambitious I'm feeling, I might add one challenging recipe to a handful of ones I feel good about. This way, I can build my confidence and expand my skills without feeling overwhelmed. If I were shopping for fifteen new ingredients in one week, I would feel overwhelmed. On the contrary, if I do one recipe with one or two new ingredients, I can get familiar with it more easily and keep making it until I become confident in it. Then as I go along, I'll find another recipe I've tagged as challenging, but it now feels much more doable because I've expanded my skillset. It's a progression that helps me feel more confident in the kitchen.

SHOPPING SYSTEMS

When you are creating new systems, consider how you can make every step of the way easier. When changing your diet, this includes shopping for your food. It is the little details that make for a good or bad experience. When you are shopping, open up your reusable bags in your cart and fill them as you go. When you get to the checkout stand, all you have to do is gently dump your bags onto the belt. This saves so much time and doesn't take any extra effort.

I have a reusable wine bag with built-in dividers so the wine bottles don't clink. I don't drink wine, but this is the perfect bag for organizing the different kinds of mesh and other grocery bags I use. It keeps everything accessible and organized and makes shopping zero waste way more attainable.

I remember one day when I was trying to use all my mesh bags and got to the bulk section. I had to switch around what items were in what bags so I had a tight enough mesh bag to use for the walnuts. That was the day I realized I needed a more organized system, and the wine bag got its purpose. I have three sections for regular-sized bags, two sections for mesh bags, one for tightly woven mesh bags (for nuts, grains, and seeds in the bulk section), and one for fruits or vegetables. The last section is for recycled paper bags.

Use reusable grocery bags and get rid of any excuses for not using them. Don't say, "I will remember next time." Get uncomfortable. Push your cart off to the side and run out to your car to get the reusable bags. Be that hilarious person carrying a stack of stuff in your arms and dropping something every few steps. Getting uncomfortable is what will help you remember. When I first started using reusable bags, there were so many times when Dakota would be standing in the checkout line, and I would be racing to the car to get our bags. And guess what? We didn't have that problem for long. It will only take a few times before you start remembering.

There are so many good options for reusable bags now. They make cute key chain ones so you can keep one in your purse or on your keys. When you make an unexpected stop, you'll never be without a bag.

Even if I don't have my handy organizer bag, I almost always have a reusable bag on hand. If for some reason, I don't have my bags with me, I still refuse to use the plastic ones. I know I might be making the cashier's day a little more complicated, so I am extra nice to them as I roll my ten apples down the conveyor belt. I'm okay with facing the uncomfortable. It's not punishment. It's a commitment.

When I start putting my items on the conveyor belt, I say right away that I don't need any plastic bags. More often than not, a cashier will begin to put my items in a plastic bag anyway. I kindly remind them with a smile, "Oh, I don't need a bag." They usually respond with something like, "Whoops. I think you already told me that." I lightheartedly say something about muscle memory and thank them for their help.

I know some people get a little nervous to be direct. Then they find it even harder to say something a second time. In a situation like this, some people might be tempted to take plastic bags to avoid discomfort. Just make eye contact, say their name, and smile. You'll probably end up being one of their best customers.

GARDENING

Gardening is a great way to have easy access to nutritious food. It is also a way to build a deeper and more meaningful connection to your food.

My year of rest is what inspired me to start a garden. I wanted to fill my days with meaningful and enjoyable activities. I have found such joy and excitement in cooking with what we are growing. The same vegetable at the store might be just as good for me, but I have put a lot more time and effort into the one I grew in the garden, and I value it more. The emotions that come with growing food, preparing it, and eating it make it more sacred.

Jesus meets me in the garden daily. Gardening is fulfilling across the board, but especially because we were made to be in nature. I have this overwhelming feeling that God had a bigger plan when He designed food to grow from the ground. He designed it not just to provide nourishment for our bodies but also for our souls. He invites me to do meaningful, present, peaceful, grounded, soul-fulfilling work. It is therapy, joy, and provision. It is security and abundance. It is awe-inspiring. It is ever-changing.

MEAL PLANNING

Do you ever feel like it takes you just as long to pick what to make as it takes to make it? Do you feel like thinking about it is more exhausting than doing it? Have you ever settled for something simple or boxed because it is easier? When you meal plan, you are giving yourself the best chance of success. You don't have to wonder what will be for dinner. You're ensuring you don't have to make decisions when you're tired. The decision has already been made for you. All you have to do is put one foot in front of the other.

For most of my life, cooking felt so daunting. I didn't understand how someone could get excited about making food look pretty. You know that saying, "Some people live to eat. Some people eat to live"? I am the second one. After going through my health journey and year of rest, I now experience food like I haven't ever before. Learning to cook what I feel good about eating has flipped my world. When I am prepping a meal, I'll often find myself caught in thankfulness. I'm thankful for the new skills I am growing. I'm thankful for the way I've changed my eating habits. I'm thankful for a healthier body and thankful that I feel more whole. I'm thankful that I feel more connected and thankful I feel proud of the way I eat. I'm thankful to be more present.

There are many ways to meal plan, but there are a few methods I have found especially helpful. The beautiful thing is you can mix and match. You can do the work as frequently or infrequently as you want. This first option is great if you are new to meal planning. You simply list out the days of the week with a general idea for your meal:

Monday: Spaghetti
Tuesday: Salad
Wednesday: Mexican
Thursday: Soup
Friday: Burgers and fries
Saturday: Chinese
Sunday: Crockpot

This way leaves more room for creativity and gives gentle direction. When I have a lot of extras in my fridge I don't know what to do with, instead of doing a specific grocery shopping trip, I'll work off this type of simple menu and use up whatever we have.

This second way of meal planning is more involved and requires more intentional planning. This option is best for when you have the time and energy and want to get creative.

First, you choose the recipes you want to make for the week. I try to have four or five meals planned and then have leftovers or wing it a few nights. This works for our family because I enjoy the simplicity of leftovers, and my husband enjoys making food with what we have on hand. Then, you make one grocery list for all those week's meals. When I am making a grocery list, I write only the ingredients I still need to buy. If I know I have one green pepper in the fridge, and the recipe calls for three, I'll only put two green peppers on the list.

If I'm trying to stick to a budget, I'll only get what is on my list, and I'll still have everything I need. If we are having a barbecue and I want to make a veggie tray, or there's a vegetable my family likes to snack on, I might get a few more than what's on my list. No matter what, I know the minimum amount I need to buy.

When I get home, I wash my produce and divide the ingredients for each meal into their own bin. I'll put a note card in the bin that has the name of the meal, the book it can be found in, and the page number. I like being able to refer to the actual cookbook because I often use shortcuts when I copy down the recipes. If you make these note cards for each meal, eventually you'll have a collection of cards that make up your own personalized recipe book. Create a filing system for your note cards so they can be reused.

I love this system. When I am ready to make a meal, I don't have to worry that we used the pepper for something else or if we will be missing a lemon. Depending on how much prep you want to do upfront, the measurements could all be done too. For example, if I get cilantro, and each meal only needs a tablespoon's worth, I can divide the cilantro into what the meals call for and then put the rest into undesignated drawers. By the time I get to cooking the meal, all I have to do is throw it together and follow the directions, which are super easy to find because of the note card already with the ingredients.

Meal planning has improved more than just my family's diet. In my first few months of meal prepping, I was shocked by how much less food waste we had. I love that we're utilizing every last bit of food and not letting anything go to waste. We aren't always running to the store because we need this one thing to make our meal. Each bit of food we buy has a designated purpose, and we are eliminating the nightly tension of trying to figure out what to make for dinner. I'm making dinner more often because I don't have to rely on my husband to get creative with what we have. Even though he is a natural cook, I don't want to put all the responsibility on him. Meal planning has boosted my confidence in the kitchen.

If you enjoy this second style of meal planning, you can take it to the next level by creating templates for a week's worth of meals. Each template has five meals, and the ingredients for those meals are condensed into one grocery shopping list. Write the book and page number of each recipe at the top of the grocery list. You can make as many of these templates as you want. Once you've made your templates, they are available for you anytime you want a plan. There are seasons where this may be more helpful to you. You don't have to make a new grocery list to make sure you have everything. You just get to pick what meals sound good and grab the list.

Steps to be done once:

1. Pick five recipes.
2. Make a grocery shopping list. Put every item on there, even if you have something in your cupboard now. If you're ever out of that item, you'll already have it on your list. Before you leave to shop, highlight what you already have at home so you know you don't need that item this time.
3. Make note cards with the book and page number of each recipe. Write this information on the grocery list as well.

Steps that need to be done every time you use the meal template:

1. Go grocery shopping.
2. Wash all of your produce.
3. Have five bins for five different meals.
4. Put all ingredients for each meal in their designated bins with the corresponding reference card.

Now, enjoy the ease of prepared meals. I am feeling pumped just writing this because I know what life-changing potential this has. I can picture some of you with your head in your hands, wondering how you'll pull this off. If you want to change your life, you just have to start somewhere. Making a plan can help guide you into bigger change. Find a way to do the work.

ACTION:

1. Identify three of your go-to snacks. What are the foods that make you feel like you have all you need?

2. Consider whether you need to replace any of these go-to snacks with a healthier alternative. If so, try one of those healthier alternatives this week.

3. The next time you forget your reusable grocery bags, don't let yourself off the hook. Run back to the car or carry your groceries in your arms. Do whatever it takes to stop using plastic bags.

4. Commit to at least one week of meal planning and make it attainable for you. Remember, it can be as easy as having a theme for each night of the week.

ORGANIZING YOUR HOME

One of the best ways to create an environment and home you love is by organizing it. It is a way to get rid of the things that have become a burden and prioritize the items you value most. That doesn't mean it's easy, especially when you're deciding what to get rid of and what to keep.

You might think that because organizing is my strength, I don't understand how difficult it can be. I want to assure you I know the struggle. I've also learned the tricks needed to get past the roadblocks. I have overcome those roadblocks myself and walked others through them. If you try to do it alone, they are harder to overcome. It helps to have someone encouraging you to stick through the uncomfortable feelings and reminding you it will be worth the peace of mind you have on the other side.

Imagine a parent at the park with their kid, encouraging them to run across one of those wobbly bridges. To the child, it feels scary, but the parent holds their hand as they walk across. After a few times, the child is doing it all by themselves. This is how I feel about organizing. I am here to tell you where to start and give you direction. I'll break it down into bite-sized instructions. In the past, when I've cleaned and organized for a client, there's always been a point when I could hand off pieces of the project to the client. Pretty soon, they were doing it themselves. Most things seem less scary when you have someone guiding you, especially someone who has confidence in the end result.

One of my rules for organizing is to make the easiest decision next. It seems like a simple concept, but how often do we look at a big, daunting task, paralyzed because we don't know where to start? We get stuck because we don't know how to move forward. Everyone seems to have a space in their home they are especially intimidated by. We're not happy with it, but we shut the door instead of dealing with it. We have good intentions to resolve the problem soon, but every time we open the door, the same thing happens.

When you find yourself in this cycle, focus on making the next easiest decision. Everyone will find resistance in different places, but if you can say to yourself, "Make the next easiest decision," you'll have your next step. It is so often the little decisions that are the biggest roadblocks. As you progress, the same task that looked so monstrous in the beginning will soon become the next easiest thing. The progress will sneak up on you.

People get stuck when they look at a task as a whole. It is big and scary to even think about doing all of it. So don't think of it like that. Look at the next easiest thing, and you will be done before you know it.

THE NINE-BIN ORGANIZING SYSTEM

Everything in your house needs a home. If something doesn't have a logical home, get rid of it or give it a home. There shouldn't be anything sitting around your house that doesn't have an allocated spot. That is how clutter happens. When you have a system in place, picking up can be done every day. If everything has a home, picking up should take ten minutes or less because you are simply putting things back in their place. You're not having to make any decisions, and it becomes muscle memory.

I have organized my home and many other people's homes in many different ways over the years. The nine-bin organizing system is my favorite. It's my most simple and uniform way to organize. This system doesn't cover every item in your home, but it does cover what I have found to be the most universal categories. Here are the nine different categories:

- Electronics
- Documents
- Projects/to fix
- Gifts
- Gift bags/tissue paper

- Extra organizing bins/baskets
- Extra disposables
- Get rid of
- Other

With this system, I'm confident I'll be able to find whatever I'm looking for in one of the first three places I check.

Everything in the same category should fit in the same space. For example, all your electronics should fit in one place. If something doesn't fit, you need to get rid of something or find a different home for that category.

ELECTRONICS

This should be the place for anything that needs power or goes to something that does. This is the spot for extra batteries, chargers, remotes, speakers, CDs, etc. This is also where you should put any tools that come with a specific device and are only used for that item. It's incredible what can fit into a square-foot bin.

I keep folders for directions and warranties in my document section. This would be an example of maybe having to check more than one category. If you are hanging onto a box for something electronic, you might leave the paperwork inside of it. The papers could be in the electronics box or in a documents folder. It is still clear that they will be in one of these two places.

DOCUMENTS

Having your documents in order can save so much hassle, time, and worry.

First, I set aside a manila folder for each company I have paperwork for. I put the logo of the company on the folder to show which papers go where. The logo is usually printed on the envelopes and documents they send. I like this system of labeling because my brain likes colors and pictures. It might be helpful to organize them alphabetically, but what works for me is organizing by category. I have my categories in clusters. The main clusters are monthly bills, cars, medical, and personal. Monthly bills are things like the mortgage, water, electricity, phone, and internet, for example.

I like getting paper statements. It has helped me out more than once, and I am way more comfortable when I have information physically in front of me. This won't be everyone's style, but here is why I like it:

1. If there is something out of sorts, I am more likely to catch it when I am physically putting the document in its place every month. I don't even really inspect the papers, but I have a mental log just from glancing them over as I put them away.
2. I have all the information I need in one place. I like being able to flip through quickly and see what the cost was the previous month or if something has changed. I prefer having a paper trail over searching my emails.
3. For me, probably the most valuable thing is that any time I make a call to customer service, I have a document right in front of me I can refer to. It makes me confident I am relaying accurate information. I can explain exactly what I'm seeing and where I'm finding it. I have their verbiage and exact numbers in front of me.
4. It gives me a place to take notes. Then I have the information I need with the right documents. Everything is in the same spot instead of on multiple notes in different places. You don't have to look any further than the paper you're going to be looking at anyway. This is a great way to document every bit of information.

When making a call to customer service, I always write down the name of the person as soon as they introduce themselves. I write the date and time I called. If for some reason the issue wasn't resolved during the call, when I call again, I have all the information I need. This increases my chance of getting the help I'm looking for.

Go through your documents once a year. I do this at the same time we do our taxes. It is a fitting time to take out the things we no longer need. I often save something just in case, and by the time I see it again, it is outdated and ready to be recycled.

Each person in my house has their own file for important documents. These are personal documents that only pertain to them. Each of our cars has its own file. They contain the title and the receipts for any work that's been done on them. Each company we pay bills to has its own file. These hold all the statements for that specific company. I have an instructions file. This is for any paperwork or instructions that came with something we bought. I have a separate warranty file. I have an ongoing tax file each year. If we get donation receipts or W2 slips, they go into that file.

PROJECTS/TO FIX

This is a place for all small projects. These might be things that need a hot glue gun, a button, or some sewing. I love this basket because I so dislike having broken things sitting around the house. I need a place for them to go, or I will end up throwing them away. When I do get out the hot glue gun, I can fix ten things instead of just fixing one.

GIFTS

This is a handy box to keep on hand for planned and spontaneous gift-giving. You know how events tend to sneak up on you, and then you find yourself frantically buying the first thing that works? The gift box eliminates this stress. The amazing thing is that I always seem to have something that's just right for the person I need a gift for. There are certain items I'll always buy when I find them because they are a good gift for anyone! Then there are the items I find when cleaning out my house. They are new, but I know I don't want to keep them. Instead of donating them, I'll put them in the gift box. No matter what time of year it is, when I see something that would make a perfect gift for someone specific, I get it. By doing this, I often get great deals. Then I save them for a special occasion. I save a lot of money shopping for gifts this way.

Some people will always buy things on sale at the end of the season and hang on to them until the appropriate season or holiday. I'm not opposed to that; the risk is these gifts can end up being less personal. No matter what time of year, there's always the potential to find the perfect thing for someone.

Although I mentioned that I save a lot of money using this system, not everyone does. It ends up being more expensive for some people because they buy gifts endlessly. Maybe they give in quantity over quality. One personal gift means more than five generic gifts. So be mindful that you don't get carried away trying to fill the gift box. It should serve as a place to put the gifts when you find them.

GIFT BAGS/TISSUE PAPER

I recycle everything. I want to emphasize this is not a place you should try to fill up. A problem I often see is that people will know they have something but can't find it. They purchase another one, only to find the original one a day later. This is inviting chaos. This space can be a home for those reusable supplies so they don't get thrown away. I have found that people are more likely to reuse items like this if they know exactly where it will go and it doesn't feel like clutter.

Make systems to make recycling easy. The way I see it, you are saving in multiple ways. You are saving the bag from the garbage. You are saving the resources you would have spent to buy the item new. In the big picture, you are helping save the item from being in demand on the market.

EXTRA ORGANIZING BINS/BASKETS

Sometimes people are concerned about the cost of all the bins and supplies they will need to get in order to organize. I can almost guarantee everything you need is already in your house. As you organize and get rid of things, you will naturally find yourself with empty containers. Even if you don't get rid of anything, just by organizing, the bins and boxes seem to appear. Don't try to make them fit just anywhere. Set them aside for now. There will be the perfect purpose for it. Don't invent uses for things that will end up cluttering your space. Wait and use it strategically.

This section can also be for small cardboard boxes or other random containers that may be recyclable but could also be great for organizing. Small, thick boxes like the boxes from new phones are the perfect size for a bathroom drawer or miscellaneous drawer.

Don't let this space overflow. Manage it, and if you need to get rid of something, do it.

Give yourself permission to have this space. Having this space helps me be more organized. Like with the gift bags, it is saving me in multiple areas. I don't have to go out and buy a new bin every time I need one. I'm not getting rid of something I can use again. I'm helping the planet by recycling and creating less demand in the market for new containers.

EXTRA DISPOSABLES

There was a point when I tracked how much of each disposable item our family used. I made a spreadsheet and bought all the disposables at the beginning of the year. I felt confident that we were well-organized and weren't making any special trips to the store for one item like deodorant or toothpaste.

When we had a new baby, and each outing took more effort, I realized that despite this system, we were still making so many random trips for just one item.

Whether you plan a year in advance or grab extras when something is on sale, make a spot for your disposable products that are backups for what is in use to avoid these random trips.

Use only one of each item at a time. Whether it's a hair tie, lip balm, deodorant, or candle, use it until it's gone, then open another one. It's common for people to buy something new, and instead of looking forward to using it while finishing up the last one, they open the new item right away. This is how things end up getting wasted. The last one never gets finished. The old one gets shoved in a drawer because it's not garbage, but we end up throwing it away anyway the next time we purge because it is old. We often keep less track of both of them as well.

This box also helps you eliminate unnecessary decision-making. You pick your favorite toothpaste and buy five of them. Whenever you need more, your decision has already been made.

GET RID OF

Everyone should always have an ongoing get-rid-of space. Have you ever been picking up around your house, and you look at the thing in your hand and think (or say out loud, let's be real), "I don't want this"? If there is not an appropriate place for it to go, it ends up back in the cupboard or toy bin. This is how our spaces can weigh us down. It is the simple fact of knowing there is stuff in our house we don't want. You'll feel better living in a space where you've intentionally chosen everything you want there.

When your get-rid-of box is full, donate it. Over time, you won't feel so frantic to get rid of things. It is a continual process.

If you are on the fence about something, try throwing it in the get-rid-of box and see if after a month you miss it. Try not to take stuff back out of this box on a regular basis, but there have been a few times I've been glad I didn't donate something immediately.

OTHER

This category is for you to designate. Each household has different patterns, rhythms, and priorities. Pick a category you would use regularly. This should be the type of space you'll add to frequently or need something from often. Use it for what makes sense for your family.

RETURN-TO-OTHERS BASKET

One of my favorite tricks for keeping my house in order is to have a return basket. It sits on our entryway bench. It makes it so easy as I am running out the door to grab the thing that belongs to the person I'm meeting or at a place I'll pass. This is important to me because I don't want to have other people's things in my house.

This is what happens with some people: You borrow a container and have the best intentions to give it back. It gets washed and sits on the counter. One day, you are in a rush packing snacks. You can't find the snack bag, but you spot the container on the counter. In a flurry, you think, "I'll just use it today." Pretty soon, this has happened three times, and instead of landing on the counter, it gets thrown in the cupboard because your husband unloaded the dishwasher and didn't know it belonged to Susy. I want to get things back to their rightful owner, and I don't want a bunch of mismatched odds and ends.

On the flip side, when I let anyone borrow something, I do it with the expectation of never seeing that thing again. I only let people "borrow" what I am willing to lose forever. Having loose ends and trying to get something back is not restful for me. I don't like thinking about who has what of mine and when they were supposed to return it. When is the appropriate amount of time before I ask for it back? How much effort do I put into retrieving it?

I keep a whole library of books that are duplicates of the ones I like. These are the ones I share. Then, I can share without giving my copy away. If they do return the book, then lovely, someone else can read it, but I don't want to rely on that. If I'm taking something to someone in a tote bag or basket, I make sure they're also items I'm okay with not getting back.

I make my best effort to return other people's things, and I loan with the mindset I might never get those items back.

I also use the return-to-others basket to store things like plastic packing material or used ink cartridges, things that need to get dropped off at the proper location. These are the kinds of items that if they didn't have a home, they'd probably end up in the garbage after I moved them three different times. I also utilize this basket for little gifts I'm not saving for any special occasion. They are thinking-of-you gifts I'd like to give the next time I see someone.

This basket is a great place for the little things you want to grab on your way out the door. Everything needs a home. This is a home for the things that shouldn't have a home in your home.

ACTION:

1. What is one space in your house that seems out of control?

2. Is there one step you can take this week to get organized?

3. Get a nine-cube organizer and put together your own system.

4. If you don't already have a return-to-others basket, make one.

14

CLEANING AND BUDGETING

Alongside organizing is cleaning. Cleaning goes hand in hand with organizing to make your home a place where you can find joy and rest.

Cleaning shouldn't be something that takes over your life. It is something that should be shared in any living situation with roommates, spouses, or children. I know it can take effort to get the family on board. It is a very valuable team activity, though. Clear expectations are key. Each person having designated tasks is helpful. We maintain throughout the week, and one day a week, we clean the whole house. We generally spend about forty-five minutes to one hour cleaning, and the main floor we clean is about 1,500 square feet. My goal is to show you how this can become attainable for you as well.

You can modify these steps and make them fit for you but do schedule the time and make the systems that will allow you to reach your goals. You might have to be a bit stricter throughout the week to make your cleaning all fit into an hour on a weeknight. When I was doing the cleaning on my own during naptime, I would set a timer for four fifteen-minute increments. I had fifteen minutes to do the initial pickup, fifteen minutes to clean the kitchen, fifteen minutes for the bathrooms, and fifteen minutes for the floors. Yes, I was running throughout the house. If you keep up during the week and use this time purposefully, one hour will be all you need. This one hour will also be a gauge of what needs to be better managed during the week.

First fifteen minutes:

This is your time to pick up things lying around the house. It's important to take this step first because it's a lot harder to clean when you're moving things or cleaning around them. So, do one big sweep. Put everything away in its home. This is where having an organizational system will make a big difference in your day-to-day life. If your house isn't that organized yet, use a basket for the things that don't have a home. This is not a decision-making time, but it will highlight what systems you need to put into place. You can do that after the house is clean. It will feel much less overwhelming to deal with the basket when the rest of the job is done. Starting with it will be a motivation zap, so just set it aside.

Second fifteen minutes:

Start cleaning the kitchen. This is usually the messiest place. Work from the top down. The best part here is when you can wipe the countertop crumbs onto the floor. Fill the dishwasher and start it. Wipe down all surfaces. Put away any machines that can be stored. Wipe the front of your appliances. Make sure the sink is empty, then wash and rinse the sink. Throw any towels or rags into the laundry pile. When you are working quickly, you will be amazed at how much you can get done in fifteen minutes, so press on.

Third fifteen minutes:

This is your time to clean the bathrooms. Again, I work from top to bottom. Start with the mirror, countertop, and sink. Everything should already be put away, so it will be a straightforward scrub. Next are toilets. I scrub the bowl first, then spray the whole thing with cleaner. I use toilet paper as my rag so I can toss it into the bowl when it is too dirty. This is an area of my life where I'd like to reduce my waste. I don't worry about the tub every week, just when it gets bad. I clean the bathroom floors separately from my regular floor routine. I have an aversion to using the same vacuum attachment I use in the bathroom around the whole house, but if this doesn't bother you, bundle it with your floor routine. I spray the floor with cleaner and use a clean rag to wipe it down.

<u>Fourth fifteen minutes:</u>

Now is the time to vacuum. Find a rhythm that works for you. I start at the front of my house and work my way back. I would rather switch attachments a few times than backtrack. If you have a different preference that works for you, run with it. Once everything is vacuumed, tuck the vacuum away and mop. I am all about steam mops and not using chemicals. The steam will kill the germs. Be careful. The steam mop can burn you. The cloths are washable, making it zero waste. The only thing you have to refill it with is water, so there is no solution to buy.

I really enjoy having a clean house. I like being able to breathe it in, even if just for a moment. I'll clean the house at the end of the day, start an oil diffuser, and just sit in my clean house. Listening to music and reading in my pristine house is one of the most relaxing ways for me to spend my time.

I know there is going to be a burnt-out mama out there who doesn't feel like this is attainable. I see your struggle. I hear you, and I encourage you to put systems in place to make it attainable. Simplify where you can and lighten the load by having others pitch in. Often, lightening the load is the best first step you can take. You can do this. There is a light at the end of the tunnel.

CLEANING THE KITCHEN EVERY NIGHT

As much as I enjoy having a clean house, it was a bumpy transition for me to start cleaning the kitchen daily.

When I first started this habit, I dreaded it. I had negative self-talk around it, and it wasn't an enjoyable part of my day. The thing was, every time I got it done, I would think, "That wasn't so bad." So why was I still having these negative thoughts about it? I was always so relieved when it was done.

I found ways to reward myself so I didn't see it as so much of a chore. Instead of watching the clock, feeling like the task was dragging on, I chose to do something that felt like a treat. I started listening to audiobooks during this time. Turning on something that captured my mind made the time pass by so quickly. I would end up feeling uplifted and refreshed instead of tense. It became an energy boost instead of a chore.

Have you heard it takes thirty days to form a habit? Train your brain to enjoy it and find ways to make it something to look forward to. Maybe you have a dance party. Maybe you open the windows and smell the fresh air. Maybe you play a show or movie or listen to a podcast. Do whatever it is you associate with relaxing or downtime.

It feels better to go to bed with a clean house. Something about having things cleaned up and put away ties up loose ends in your mind. It helps your brain rest. Have you ever had those moments where you are almost asleep, and then you jolt awake, wondering if you locked the door, turned off the light, or switched the laundry? Even if you aren't motivated enough to go resolve whatever it is, it startles you from your sleep. Our brains like closed loops.

Starting your day in a clean kitchen is a win. It creates a snowball effect of wins throughout your day. If you go into the kitchen first thing in the morning, and your thoughts every morning are positive instead of negative, think about how that will set your day up for success. Do the things today that will set you up for success tomorrow.

A QUICK BREAKDOWN OF DECLUTTERING

Decluttering is intimidating to many people. This is what I would say if I saw the blank look on your face that shows you don't know where to start.

Set yourself up for success. Get out boxes or bags for these four categories: garbage, recycling, get rid of, and move. Start with one room, and don't do anything with the bags until the room is fully clean and organized. If you try and do all the small errands in between, I can almost guarantee you'll get distracted. When you are done, it will be a super straightforward cleanup.

<u>Garbage and recycling:</u>

Collect the garbage and recycling while you are decluttering. You'll throw away any garbage at the end after the room is clean, but not yet. When the cleaning is finished, immediately take the garbage to your curbside bin and be done with it. Keep recycling in its own pile, bag, or box. Even if you find a box you might use later, don't set it aside. Put it in the recycling pile. If you grab it back out for a specific use, great, but don't start making more random piles.

Get rid of:

Put anything you no longer want in the get-rid-of box. Don't frazzle yourself thinking about if your sister might want it. Now is not the time to sort. We slow down the process and make roadblocks for ourselves when we try to make too many decisions at one time. In the end, you can sort out what you want to donate, sell, or throw away, but don't spend your brainpower on that yet.

Move:

As you sort, make a pile of items you know you want to keep but don't belong in that space. Don't worry about where to put it yet. Putting it in this pile is all you need to do for now. If you try to find a space for it at this point in the process, it will likely get moved multiple times and slow down your momentum. It will take you to other places in the house and leave tasks half-done. Stay focused.

Keep the pile right outside of the room you are decluttering. It feels good to throw things out the door. It helps you see your progress and barricades you in until you are done (ha ha!). If at any point you are feeling depleted or discouraged, look at this pile—it screams progress. Then dig back in.

Now, you can pick a space to start decluttering. I would encourage you to start small. Maybe it's a desk, a closet, or a nook. Get the first win under your belt. Start with anything that needs to be thrown away or recycled. Let go of anything that is easy for you to get rid of. It will be tempting to stop halfway through the process and put something away, especially if you know where you want it to go. Have self-control and just put it in the box.

As you clear a shelf, drawer, or surface, this is the time to wipe it down or vacuum it out. However big the section you are working in, just make sure to clean it before you put the stuff back. Now that you've sorted your items and cleaned the space, you are ready to organize. Once you have accounted for every item in the space, you can begin to put things in their home. I am a stickler about this: you have to look at every item. There are no excuses and no exceptions.

Use this system in every space in a room until the room is finished. Once everything is off the floor, the finishing touch is to vacuum. Now you have a completely clean space.

Don't be discouraged by the piles outside the door. After seeing the clean room, you should have a renewed hope and energy to push through the final steps. Usually, the success feels so good it makes the final steps easy.

Take out the garbage. It's an easy win. The get-rid-of box is next. If you want to grab anything and put it in the gift box, now is the time to do that. Then you should put the box in your car immediately. I always had a deal with my cleaning clients that I would take their donation pile with me. I knew if it sat at their front door, things would start to crawl back out. If there are things you don't want to donate, make a box of items to sell. Give yourself a time limit. If you haven't sold them by the deadline, then it is time to donate them.

Finally, there are the items you need to put back in the right places around your house. This is the most tedious task, but it should be obvious where to put things for the most part. As you get more into cleaning and organizing, everything will have a specific home, and there shouldn't be any hesitation. If you are decluttering your whole house, wait until you have organized each room to put things in their place.

Now you're done. Self-five!

BUDGETING

Before I took my year of rest, I had always worked. I had made my own money since I was six years old, and I have taken a lot of pride in that. I also know that I've misplaced my trust, safety, and identity in money and my ability to make it. Money is seeking power over our lives. It wants to be number one. It wants to be the star of the show. It wants to distract you and deceive you. The Enemy of your soul uses money for all these purposes.

How much should we spend? How much should we give? How much

time should we devote to making money? How much brain space do we give to money? These are the questions I've been struggling to answer.

God used my year of rest to change my view of money and the weight I give it. He is stripping my identity and security from money and showing me how to surrender on a whole new level. I have had to surrender control over my finances and trust in God and my husband to provide. At the beginning of my marriage, I experienced some deep wounding around money. I had built a wall to protect myself in this area of our marriage. I didn't want to get hurt in this way again, and I withheld my trust. God is asking me to take down this wall. He wants me to trust in His provision and my husband.

In the past, I saw the work I achieved and the money I earned as things done in my own power. I thanked God but felt like I had earned these things on my own. It was more of an entitled than a humble thanks. I pray that no matter where I go from here, I will always be thankful and have a humble heart. That is another beautiful part of living in our strengths and using them to glorify God. God gave you skills and talents to share with the world. He wants them to fulfill you and glorify Him, not make you prideful and self-reliant.

This year has challenged me to believe in my worth. I need to know the role I play is enough, even if it doesn't manifest monetarily. When I used to list off all the tasks, chores, and errands I had done in a day, it pointed a spotlight on my insecurity. I didn't believe being me was enough. I didn't believe my role was enough. No matter how much I advocated for other stay-at-home moms, I didn't feel like I was enough.

Our purpose in life isn't to make money. God will provide, and He wants us to stop running. Stop chasing money, and He will provide abundantly. He wants to bless us. We have to stop hustling to live in abundance. Abundance is a state of being. Someone could be making ten times as much money as you are, and you could still be living in more abundance. It is a mindset.

There are still days I have to fight to believe these things, but my life has changed drastically now that I'm not chasing my worth. My transformation isn't over, but I'm so much better at recognizing when my insecurities are telling me to run. I can identify sooner when I am running. I am choosing to be present and let the to-do list wait.

God also challenged my view of giving. When we are only focused on trying to reach our financial goals, giving feels like a setback. Through my season of rest, I found so much more joy in giving. It brought such perspective to the gifts we receive from God. When you view your resources as provision instead of pride, it is easier to give away.

All this means I now view budgeting differently. When I keep track of where my money goes, I can have more to give. I can use my money purposely to make a difference in the world. Money is power. Where you choose to spend your money gives power to that organization or corporation. The bigger an organization grows, the more power and the louder voice it has. How you spend your money has an exponential impact. You can buy a product that helps fund a mission that changes people's lives for the better. Decide what businesses you want to support, whether it is a small mom-and-pop shop or a chain store. Every time you hand over your money, you are funding some sort of agenda. Do the work to make sure you're supporting the messages you want the world to hear.

I have a simple budgeting spreadsheet that works for me. I like to reset and adjust this template every year depending on our budgeting needs for that year. Your method of budgeting doesn't have to be fancy. I did it on paper for years. Just start somewhere. Tracking is the first step to finding out what changes you need to make.

Category	Budgeted Number	Actual Number
Income	(Total income = all income with rollover included)	(The expenses subtracted from the income)
Paycheck One		
Paycheck Two		
Rollover From Previous Month	(Positive or Negative)	
Expenses	(Total outgoing)	
House	(Standard)	
Car Insurance	(Standard. If you pay six months in advance, divide the total number by six and put that amount into savings each month.)	

Phone	(Standard)	
Internet	(Standard)	
Utilities		
Water	(Add all twelve months together and divide by twelve to get a medium and accommodate high and low bills. Have a section in your bank for the rollover so it is there when there is a high bill.)	
Power	(Same as water)	
Budget	(Have a baseline based on income.)	
Groceries	(Have a standard budgeted number for groceries at the beginning of the month. At the end of the month, total the real number of all transactions.)	(Each transaction)
Gas	(Have a standard budgeted number for gas at the beginning of the month. At the end of the month, total the real number of all transactions.)	(Each transaction)
Fun	(We get cash at the beginning of the month. Have a standard number for each month.)	
Tithe	(10% of total income)	
Savings/Investing		
Variable		
Anything Unexpected and Not Budgeted		

Once you set up your template, you don't have to do it again. It is an easy way to keep ongoing and up-to-date numbers.

We had a cash budget for a long time. We still bounce back to this when we are having a hard time sticking to our budget. You think about money differently when you physically have to hand over the bills. If the money isn't physically there, you can't buy whatever it is. You can't because you don't have the money. Your decision is already made for you. I can see how a cash budget could be frustrating, but it also brings more intentionality to where you spend your money.

It might be uncomfortable, but I would recommend going cold turkey, especially if you have a big transition to make. It is better to be frustrated and on track than to be comfortable and cheat the commitment you made to yourself.

You have the willpower. You have the resources. When you see the fruit and the benefits of staying on track, you'll have the motivation to do so.

ACTION:

1. This week, choose one small area in one room to declutter using the four-bag system.

2. The next time you clean, set a timer for yourself. Make it fun and see how much you can get done in that time.

3. Identify just one room you know you want to declutter. Imagine how it would affect that space if you did. How would you feel?

4. Take some time this month to write out your budget.

15

SUSTAINABLE LIVING

So many of us wish we were living more sustainably. So why aren't we? Just like with organizing, many people end up not doing it at all because they don't know where to start.

Start with what tugs at your heart. It will be the easiest thing to change and keep doing consistently. Start with one little change. Pick the step that feels simple and attainable. That is how transformation happens. It's better to make one little change than to look at all the things you could change and never start. Do the next best thing next. Start with something that you can get excited about changing.

I can get down on myself because I know there are so many things I could be doing. When you are feeling like this, use it as an opportunity to get out a notepad and start brainstorming. Don't let those feelings drag you down. Use them to propel you forward. Once you have a list of goals for sustainable living, start to number or categorize them. Keep coming back to this list. It is amazing how much progress you can gain when you move forward inch by inch. Soon, you'll have made more progress than you ever could have imagined.

Remember to give yourself credit for the changes you've already made. You're not failing at sustainable living if you still have garbage at the end of the month. The point is to reduce your waste. It will be a process and will happen gradually. Sometimes, it might feel like you aren't doing that much, but when you look back a year from now, you'll see how all that progress has accumulated.

If you're not already stoked about living more like your great-grandparents, then get ready. To some, these methods might feel overboard.

To some, it might feel like we are only scratching the surface. No matter where you are, I hope this inspires you to take the next step.

INSPECTING YOUR GARBAGE

Knowing what items you throw away most is the first step to reducing your waste. What is in your trash? Seriously, go look in your garbage can.

When we first moved into our current house, we had a problem with mice. I *really* don't like mice. To avoid attracting the mice, I got into the habit of taking out the garbage every time I left the house. At that stage of my life with a toddler, that was two or three times a day. This was probably overkill, but I was paranoid about these critters invading our house. We had just moved into our new (110-year-old) remodeled house. I was not handling it well. Now, we have a mouse-hunting cat that has solved the problem.

I realized I didn't need nearly as big of a bag if I was taking out the trash three times a day. So, I got creative. If I finished a block of cheese, that was the garbage bag until the next time I left the house. People get plastic bags specifically to put more plastic bags in. I reversed this.

This was a revolutionary idea for me. We were going to throw this plastic away anyway. Why not put it to use and save another bag in the process? I used tortilla chip bags, cheese bags, bread bags, cracker bags, vegetable bags, and more. Every and all types of bags became garbage bags.

This was one of the first baby steps for me. I began to notice what we were throwing away. We started slowly eliminating the items that came in disposable packing. When I bought something in a package, I thought about what sustainable option I could use instead. For example, you could buy five pounds of prebagged apples or put five pounds of apples into a mesh bag. Just start noticing the little things.

EATING WELL MEANS LESS WASTE

Making shifts in your diet can also reduce waste. Once I was eating more vegetable-based meals, I purchased fewer packaged items. I felt empowered to grow the food I had previously been buying. I was eating more from the earth, and the earth makes biodegradable packaging: peels.

Changing my diet made it seem possible for me to grow my food. Before, I already had a desire to garden, but I didn't see it as a way to replace the food I was buying. I couldn't imagine it because of what I was eating. I couldn't grow cereal. I could grow zucchini, lettuce, tomatoes, and more. Once I changed what I was eating for breakfast, I saw it was possible to grow my own breakfast.

Gardening makes the most sense if you are replacing the things you would usually be buying. It's a big step to imagine what to plant in a garden when you don't eat those foods regularly. If you are eating the foods that are possible to grow, it feels more attainable. It is so encouraging to go to the store and think, "I don't have to buy that. It's growing at my house," and watch your grocery bills go down and your shopping trips become less frequent. I save gas and other resources by going to the store less often. Soon, you will see the effects of gardening in many different parts of your life.

THRIFT SHOPPING

I was raised to shop at thrift stores, although I wasn't always proud of it. There was a time when I was borderline embarrassed about it. Now, I am a proud thrifter. As I have grown and made my own path, thrifting is 100% my choice and preference. It aligns much more with my values and meshes beautifully with my lifestyle.

I like to find hole-in-the-wall thrift stores. I have found that chain stores often have higher prices. It is becoming more common for them to research the value of their items, which means higher prices. They are also taking advantage of the online market and selling anything of significant value online, not even putting it in their store. This makes it harder to get great deals.

When my husband and I lived in western Washington, I found out which stores valued which items and which items they were trying to move quickly. One store might value furniture more highly and put a high price tag on it. If you found that same piece at another store down the road, it might be worth a quarter of the cost. When I went into a thrift store, I knew which items to look for there.

At one store, I wouldn't even look at the furniture because, in my opinion, it was overpriced. I would beeline to their books because they only cost ten cents. There was a store that sold their clothes for one dollar each every Sunday. That made it easy not to look for clothes anywhere else.

Shopping at thrift stores saves waste in so many ways. The first thing that comes to my mind is the packaging. By the time you see an item in the thrift store, its packaging has already been discarded, and it doesn't get any new packaging at the thrift store. Even if I did find something in the package, I viewed it as already having been disposed of. The waste happened when the item was first bought. Oftentimes, the only waste you'll get from a thrift store item is one small tag. They'll even take the hangers back and reuse those.

So much of what is donated to thrift stores doesn't get sold, and it's sad to think about what happens to the items that don't sell. There are organizations that make their best effort to recycle everything they can, but a lot of donated items still get thrown in the dumpster. Not only are you saving packaging when you shop at a thrift store, you might be saving an item that was on its way to the dumpster.

When I am buying from a thrift store, it isn't driving production like it does when I buy something new. If you need a toaster and you can buy one at the thrift store, their records might show they sold a kitchen item, but they won't order more toasters. You can save an item from being manufactured and added into the world wrapped in packaging. If there isn't as much demand for new clothes, gadgets, home décor, etc., then it forces the manufacturers to switch gears.

It only takes one person to change the world. You have to believe what you do matters. Start somewhere. Be the change. Be the one person standing out in the collective whole. It only takes one person to start a movement. Do what you can no matter what others choose to do. Some people aren't even opposed to thrift shopping—they just have never been exposed to it. It might take an enthusiastic friend with a few good reasons to change their mind.

THE POWER OF SEWING

Today, I made two draft stoppers for our kitchen doors. My daughter called them snakes, which made me laugh. Doing this project inspired me to share my love of sewing with you. Sewing is so creative and artistic.

I love feeling empowered to use what I already have. Sewing is such a powerful skill because as long as you have the supplies, you can transform them into whatever you need.

This is one of those skills where if you learned it young, you'll always have it. I learned basic sewing in my middle school home economics class. Our first project was to make a pillow. It had nine quilt squares on the front, and the back was one big piece. Later in high school, I took more home economics classes and expanded my sewing skills. While I was still in high school, I made a full-size quilt, batting and all, for my older brother. I made it out of all his running shirts. That is the project I am most proud of to this day. I have made quilts out of my own running shirts, and I have made one for my husband with his running shirts. When you are a runner, T-shirts are a staple.

Years later, I still don't feel like I venture into anything too fancy. I did my first zipper project just last month. This month is the first time I have done a project with elastic. I have been sewing for over ten years and am just now learning these things. The basics will get you pretty far. Sewing is pretty forgiving. Depending on what you are working on, most things don't have to be perfect.

I would encourage you to find an inexpensive sewing machine. It will give you back so much more than you pay for it. Sewing machines will last a long time, or forever if you take care of them. The possibilities are endless as you grow in your skillset. It has saved me money on things I wanted to buy but could make instead, things I could fix instead of buying again, and gifts I would have bought for others but spent time on instead.

It is fairly easy to get material other people have discarded. Material scraps can often be found for free, but even if you do pay, they are much less expensive than buying new fabric. Keep using your own leftovers as well. Another thing I have done to recycle my scraps is make a "poof." This is made with any material or thread I have used to its full extent and am ready to discard. Instead of throwing it away, it gets stuffed into the "poof." (It is like a footstool. Instead of buying stuffing for it or throwing away my scraps, I use my scraps for the stuffing and save on both ends.)

I love that I can go to a market or boutique and get ideas for new projects to try. I usually snap pictures of a few things I think I could do and then experiment on my own. The possibilities are truly endless.

If no one has told you, you can learn to sew. Sewing is one of the best ways to live more sustainably. You don't have to be an expert to have confidence in the basics.

REPLACING DISPOSABLES

Think about what you throw away most often. This could go hand in hand with inspecting your garbage. Don't try to do some fancy new thing that doesn't already fit your lifestyle. There is no point in getting cute bamboo utensils if you don't eat anywhere but your house. Yes, it is sustainable and trendy, but if that isn't where the majority of your waste comes from, it won't have as big of an impact. If you eat out often and catch yourself throwing away plastic utensils and straws all the time, then go for it. Start with the things that will make the biggest impact.

You can also consider what will pay for itself first. There are some items that will just be a cute upgrade. Depending on your lifestyle though, some items can save you a lot of money. A bidet would reduce, if not eliminate, your toilet paper consumption and therefore your bill.

You can also start here: what disposable item will you run out of next? If you are like me and stock up on disposables far in advance, you can still look at what you will run out of next. If you have enough dryer sheets for a year, but your paper towels will run out next month, consider how you could replace your paper towels when they run out. This takes some of the decision-making out of which sustainable practice to try next. When you feel overwhelmed thinking about all the things you "should" be doing, just focus on the next best step next. It's a great feeling to go to the store, see an item, and think, "I don't have to buy that anymore."

When I started replacing my disposables with reusable items, I thought about what I would need most if I didn't have access to a store next week. I am talking about necessity, not convenience. Menstrual products were the biggest necessity I could think of. If I had no access to outside consumerism, I would eventually need an alternative for my menstrual products. Consider what disposable products you depend on. This is another way to measure a starting point.

There are so many ways to think about this, and different approaches will click with different people, as well as different motivators. Find the things you can get excited about so you aren't detoured by the discomfort. For some people, it will be saving money. For some people, it will be keeping garbage out of landfills. Others won't want to be dependent on our system of consumerism. Maybe you're passionate about future generations and our planet. You may have other reasons or a combination of reasons. Is your "why" big enough to be uncomfortable for?

Cloth diapers are a great example of a sustainable alternative. I spent the same amount on cloth diapers as I would have spent on two to three boxes of disposable diapers. They've already lasted me three years and are still going strong. Let's say the average person uses a box of disposable diapers every two months. Based on that vague math, it took me a maximum of six months for my investment in cloth diapers to pay itself off. (And I think that is on the conservative side for disposable diaper use.)

I also use reusable Norwex cloths to wash my face. I can buy a facial cloth that will replace face wash for the rest of my life. The goal is to buy sustainable alternatives that are good for the planet and worth the investment. Here are some replacements for disposable items:

Disposable Product	Sustainable Product
Paper napkins	Cloth napkins
Dryer sheets	Dryer balls, or even better, hang dry
Disposable diapers	Cloth diapers
Plastic bag for car garbage	Reusable garbage bag you dump at the gas station
Plastic or paper grocery bags	Reusable grocery bags
Plastic fruit/veggie bags	Mesh or drawstring bags
Plastic bags for bulk items	Tightly woven mesh bags
Toilet Paper	Bidet and cloth wipes (Okay, I know I've lost some of you here, but think about it—if you've ever used cloth diapers with your children, it is practically the same thing.)
Pads or tampons	Reusable underwear or cup
Paper towels	Small cloths
Cotton swabs	Silicone swabs
Plastic utensils	Bamboo utensils

Liquid shampoo	Shampoo bar
Liquid hand soap	Bar soap
Plastic wrap	Elastic covers
Shaving razors	Palm tweezers (If you haven't heard of this, look it up.)
Wax paper	Silicone mats

USING BUSINESS WASTE

These days, businesses are made to streamline. They bulldoze through the production of their product and leave everything else by the wayside. This results in an overproduction of one kind of waste. They have too much of the same thing and don't have the desire to market it because it's their waste. Their profitability comes from their marketed item. It would be a distraction for them to sell the waste from their specialty item. Their waste is the part they're trying to get out of the way so they can do their job.

Coffee shops are one of the first places I learned about that often give away their waste. Some places have bags of used coffee grounds you can take for free. Used coffee grounds are good for so many things such as gardening, burning to keep mosquitoes away, and making natural scrubs for your skin. Coffee shops streamline coffee. It wouldn't make sense for them to market their used grounds. They produce coffee grounds faster than they can get rid of them. Anything they can give away saves them from having to throw it away.

I'm going to put another face on it with used bookstores. They get so many books that they can't shelve them all. It costs more for them to hold on to the low-value books than to dispose of them. It costs them money in terms of the floor space they could be using for high-value books.

Start thinking about the businesses you go to. What is their waste? Oftentimes, they will give it to you for free. It's either that or they have to pay to dispose of it. These are some of my favorite resources: burlap bags from coffee roasters, coffee grounds from local coffee shops, and pallets from industrial businesses. I haven't utilized this one yet, but you can feed animals with the spent grain from breweries. There are so many great things being thrown away, and they are waiting right there for you to use them.

YOU WILL MAKE MISTAKES, AND THAT'S OKAY

This weekend was an exhilarating and exhausting one on our farm. Today, we homed everything that had relocated to our house in the last two days. I am so thankful for my kind neighbor who spent his afternoon helping me move my bees into their hive boxes. As much as I like to think I would have done fine on my own, this was my first time moving the bees, and it was nice to have a little assurance that everything would be done right.

With a three-year-old and a puppy to consider, the plan was to do the transfer when everyone was napping. It didn't turn out that way, so I ended up having lots of helpers. Kennedy has a homemade beekeeper's suit, and it was so fun seeing her wear it. She was telling me how thankful she is that we have bees at our house but that she wasn't sure she wanted to be outside with them. In the end, both baby and puppy did so well, and we transferred the bees in less than twenty minutes.

I am so excited that the thing I've been waiting for and prepping for over a year is finally here. I am really doing this.

At the same time, we are moving forward with our farm and finding new ways of sustainable living. We are also making plenty of mistakes. I have lost two batches of chicks in an incubator now. I am confident my next time will be successful.

It is okay to mess up. Messing up isn't failing. This is a concept I am still learning. I make better projects with recycled materials because I give myself more freedom to make mistakes. I used to get so worked up about measuring the wrong length and wasting a piece of material with a wrong cut that I wouldn't even want to do the project. I used to measure everything out and have Dakota make the cuts. It took me a while to realize it wasn't because I was scared of the saw but scared of making an undoable mistake. I was afraid to make a move too soon. I was paralyzed.

As I learn more about myself, I've realized that I learn by doing. Even if that means making a big mess or "wasting" material, I need to learn hands-on. I have learned to let it be part of the process. It is more rewarding for me to have a big mess and make some mistakes than to have a perfect product but be nervous the entire time I am making it. I feel so much more empowered, do a better job, and actually make fewer mistakes when I can let the pressure go. I am learning to accept the imperfect process.

As you start to make changes and bring new systems into your life, you will make mistakes. Maybe you try to meal plan and end up eating fast food instead. Maybe you start to organize a room and leave the project unfinished. Maybe you commit to cleaning the kitchen every night, and one night you just don't have the energy. Maybe you buy something new when you want to be thrifting. Don't let the fear of failing stop you from even trying in the first place. Let go of the idea you have to be perfect. None of your efforts will be wasted. Change will take time and many, many mistakes. In the middle of your mistakes, you will find glimmers of progress and success.

With my first batch of chicks, I didn't realize the eggs were only viable for seven to ten days after being laid. I thought they could last months. That's not true for hatching. Nonetheless, I followed through with the whole cycle just in case any were viable, but we didn't have any signs of life. The second batch I chilled. I am so sad to say ironically on Easter. We were headed out for our Easter celebrations, and I gave the chicks water to keep the humidity in their incubator up. In my hustle, I didn't get their lid back on all the way. When we got back, I found the lid misplaced. At that point, I wasn't counting on any of the eggs hatching but continued the cycle with a week remaining. When I heard cheeps on the twentieth night, I was so excited. It was such an incredible experience. Life was being created in my living room. An animal was forming in a shell that most of us have only experienced as breakfast.

It is truly incredible how much our space has changed in a year. Our whole front yard is lined with crates that are being used as raised garden beds. The crates are trellised for vertical growth as well. In our side yard, I am using pallets as shallow raised beds for lettuce. I also have a narrow raised bed for beans and peas. This one side of my house gets the most shade and has worked so well for growing lettuce. The backyard has both a large and small animal coop, trellises, crates for raised beds, fruit trees, a greenhouse, and more. I had no idea how much we could do with our space. The more I learn, the more I realize what we can do.

This progress was possible because we committed to keep trying and keep making mistakes. If you want to make a change, just start somewhere. A year from now you'll look back and be amazed by the progress you see.

ACTION:

1. What change toward sustainability do you most want to make? What is tugging at your heart in this moment? What is one step you can take this week to make that change?

2. Take a moment to inspect your garbage, even if it is just a small can. What stands out to you?

3. The next time you need a new clothing item, see if you can find it at a thrift store first.

4. Choose one of the disposable items from the list above. The next time you need that item, try switching to a reusable version.

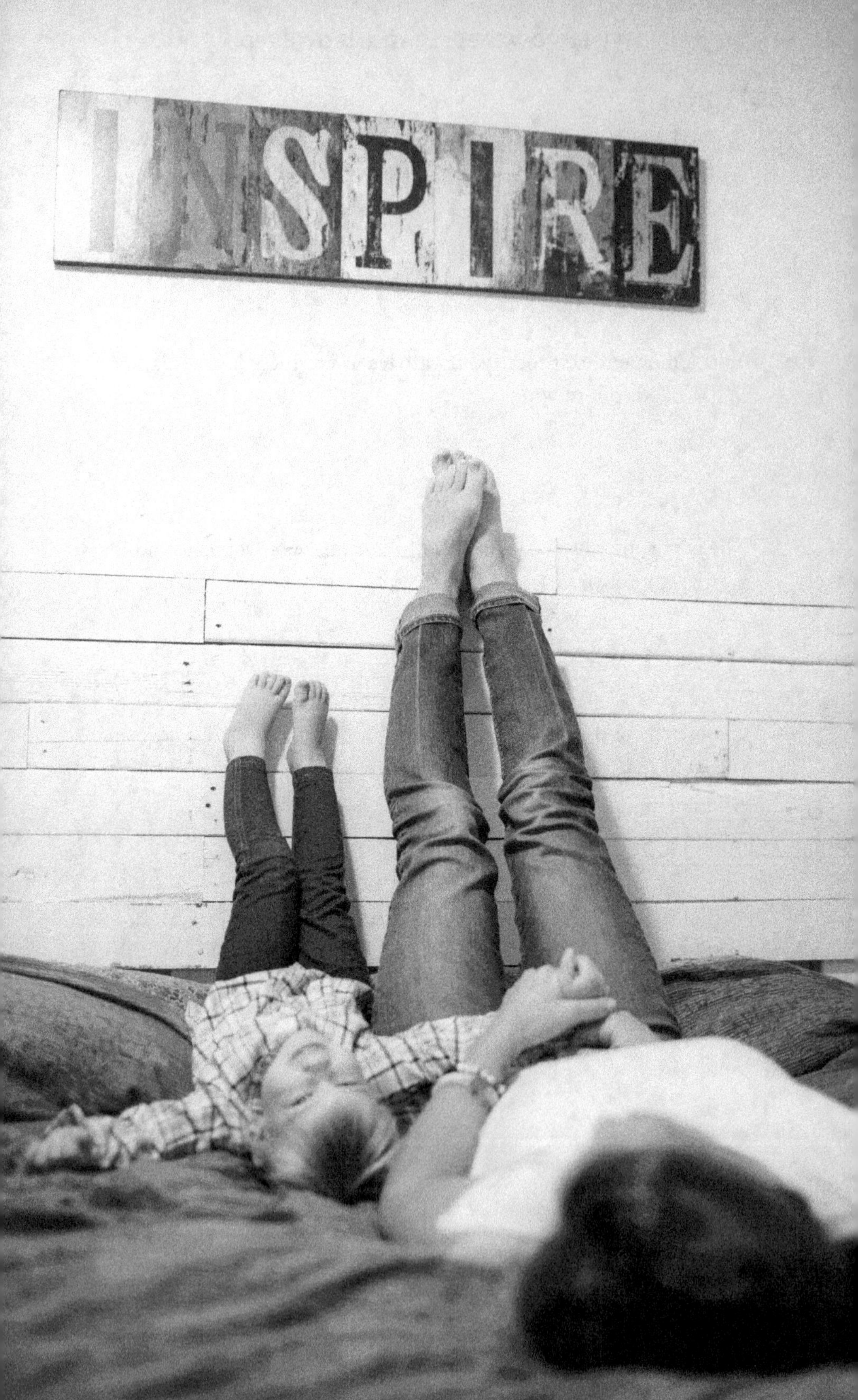
INSPIRE

CONCLUSION

You may feel hesitant to try things you haven't done before. The key to this journey is to take baby steps. We live in a culture of instant gratification, and baby steps might feel unrewarding at first. I can get tripped up by thoughts that I'm not doing enough. I criticize myself before other people can. In the past, I have quit too soon. Don't. Just focus on the next step.

I took gymnastics when I was younger, and they had raised balance beams. I learned that to get across, I just needed to keep taking the next step. Elite gymnasts aren't looking at the crowd or their coaches. They are focused on the next step. If you stretch out too far, you risk injuring yourself instead of making progress.

If we wait around for the perfect time or conditions to change our lives, then we'll never make progress. We'll become people who had good intentions but never changed. Hold yourself accountable. Don't just dream of a better life—reach for it. Each month, write down three steps you can take toward the lifestyle you wish you had. Put them somewhere you'll see them often. Once you start making progress, it will become so much easier to keep making it. As you live more and more in the lifestyle you want, you will gain confidence and pride, and it will become even easier to make the next step. Keep taking baby steps.

LOOK FURTHER

For so long, I felt like I had to do everything in one day. Now, I make a list of goals for the month and am amazed at how much I actually get done. It feels like I am doing less but getting more accomplished. Did you hear that? Read it again. Sometimes doing less in a more focused way makes a bigger difference. That is the key to long-term thinking. It doesn't always seem to make sense, but I am so thankful this is how it works. It is the upside-down kingdom.

I used to get caught up in judging how much someone else was doing. It has been a journey, one that is still in progress, to stop judging other people's journeys. I was always drawn to people who were doing a lot because I thought that meant they had their lives figured out. When I was running a hundred miles an hour, it didn't make sense for me to look to someone who was walking leisurely. My heart was hard in judgment because I thought they weren't working hard enough. Really, they were probably making more progress, with less pain, than I was. It's like getting your car unstuck from the mud or snow. If you've ever been in this scenario, you know you have to press the gas down slowly to get traction. If you stomp on the gas, you only dig in deeper. Sometimes, slowing down makes us more effective.

We can get so discouraged when we think things aren't happening fast enough. We live in a time when the world is constantly trying to do more and do it faster. When we look at the big picture, we feel more freedom to set aside the hustle. When we are firm in our purpose and direction, we don't need to prove to the world that we are trying. We get better results when we commit for the long run and let the journey take its course.

For most of my life, I didn't feel satisfied until I had completed a task. What I found was that I was never satisfied. I was always striving. When I was so caught up in reaching the finish line, I missed the journey. When I was grinding to get to the end, most of my life was misery for occasional moments of victory. Then, I'd reenter the cycle just as soon as I'd completed it.

I was missing the bigger picture. I was missing who I was becoming. I chose achieving over becoming who I truly wanted to be. I am amazed by how I've grown since I decided to open my hands and submit to the journey God has for me. The world shouts that you need to keep achieving more and more. Striving for this type of achievement isn't living in fullness. When you are living in fullness, you will still achieve and reach your goals, but the pace and gentleness may be confusing as it is contrary to the world. It looks different this way. It feels way different. It is far more fulfilling.

Keep some short-term goals, but make sure they align with the long-term, and then let the hustle fall by the wayside. When you are living in confidence about the purpose of your journey, you will be so much less tempted to overpack today, this month, or this year. When you rest in God's perfect plan for your life and pursue growth, live with open hands, and trust God's timing, you will feel free to live in your strength and be used powerfully right where you are.

SHARE WHAT YOU HAVE

There will always be people who are ahead of you in your journey. There will always be people who are behind you. I have one neighbor whom I have been learning gardening and beekeeping from for a few summers now, and I have one neighbor who just got her first three chicks.

I often don't feel like an expert. I know there are people out there who have way more knowledge and experience than I do. I worry about coming off like I know more than I do. I feel like a baby learner in so many areas and often feel unqualified to share what I do know. I'm learning to share what I have no matter where I am in life. What you have to share is valuable.

Don't look around to confirm there is someone else with more expertise than you. Look up to them. Keep learning and then turn to the people who can learn from you. No one can share or create in the unique way you can. No one can present it quite like you. Often, people are actually more receptive when the gap between you doesn't feel so big. If the gap is too big, people might disqualify themselves. They are too intimidated by how "far behind" they are. It wouldn't make sense to ask the president about your city or state politics. Oftentimes, we don't need help from the president. We need help from the city council.

You have something valuable to share. There is someone who wishes they knew what you did and could benefit from what you have inside of you.

Sometimes, I don't feel like I have the credibility to share what I'm learning because I haven't been "successful" at it yet. I had the experience of going on a walk with a friend who had no experience with beekeeping and didn't know even the basic terms. So, I explained. At that moment, I surprised myself with how much I actually did know. By sharing our knowledge with others, we affirm what we know and find where the gaps in our knowledge are.

We don't have to arrive at the finish line to be effective. I have news for you. We won't ever arrive. I used to have so much resistance to taking the next step because I didn't feel qualified, but Mark Batterson says it powerfully, "God doesn't call the qualified; God qualifies the called."[34]

It is not where you are on the journey. It is that you are on the journey. Just be on the journey. Don't let anything keep you from sharing what you have.

ONE YEAR

My one-year challenge changed me so much. When my year of rest began, one year felt like such a long time. I didn't know if I could do it. I asked God if He was really asking me to do this or if I was making things up. I was hesitant because it was so out of my comfort zone. I thought maybe I could slow down or change focus, but I couldn't. I gained perspective by having the comfort and security of work stripped away. I would have missed the purpose if I'd tried to do this halfway.

I have always been competitive. I was the kid who wouldn't play if I didn't believe I could win. I wanted certainty and control. God has been asking me to hand that over. He has been asking me to take the next step, even though I don't know the end result. He is asking that of all of us. I know God wants to use each of us in really big ways. For God to use me in a bigger way, I had to stop running and surrender. I had to let go of the results and keep being obedient to God no matter the outcome.

The journey hasn't been easy. I have felt big emotions, discomfort, and the desire to soothe the pain, all the while knowing deep in my soul that this pain is temporary if I choose to walk with Jesus through it. He would only ask me to walk this road if it led to more of Him. The road has been painful, but I so desperately want more of Jesus, and I have hope for where the road ends. I once heard someone use the example of the Israelites walking in the desert for forty years. If they had been rescued early, they would have missed out on the lessons God had for them. God doesn't want us to be in pain, but He won't let any pain go to waste.

---

[34] Batterson, *The Circle Maker,* 78.

There were moments during my season of rest when I thought the pain would break me. At one point, I had such an intense spiritual moment. I felt Jesus give me the option to go home. It shook me deeply. I cried and prayed and decided to fight. At that moment, I asked God, "Who am I supposed to be fighting for?" He answered me with specific people. At that moment, I chose to fight for this life. I chose to fight to stay here. I can't help but crack a smile as I write this because I know this is going to be a little overly spiritual for some people, but this is for the people who need a wake-up call. We weren't designed to just make it through this life. We were designed to live passionately with a mission and a calling. So, ask God who you are supposed to be fighting for. Ask Him what you are supposed to be fighting for.

This book is for the people who have a hill to climb. There is work to do. There always will be. I have sometimes wondered if there are people who don't have a hill to climb, or if they only have a molehill, not a mountain. I have decided the answer is no. Everyone has a mountain to climb. Some people may be better equipped. Maybe they had parents, coaches, teachers, and leaders in their life that helped guide them. So maybe they can go further faster. We all have obstacles and uphill battles. This is just part of the journey, and it is how we will get stronger.

It is always risky to go somewhere big. Your path will have unknowns. We don't get anywhere big without facing our fears. To everyone, that "somewhere big" is going to look different, and if you compared it to someone else's, you would be cheating yourself. It has taken me a long time to rest in the fact that only I can measure if I'm doing my best. My best might disappoint you, or it might blow your socks off. For so many years, I froze because I couldn't handle not knowing if I was meeting other people's expectations. My worth was based on my accomplishments and other people's reactions. I am still in progress, but I no longer have to be the best at everything I do. I can laugh a little more. I can be a little sillier and give myself more grace when something doesn't turn out how I envisioned it. I love the idea from Mark Batterson that "God always recycles our mistakes."[35]

God took me on a journey in writing this book. I didn't know what would happen with this book, and at one point, I suggested to my husband

---

[35] Batterson, *The Circle Maker*, 64.

that maybe it was a journey just for me. I didn't really need to publish it, did I? This was me resisting my calling, and the Holy Spirit quickly kicked that idea to the curb. This book was a step of obedience for me. I couldn't stop short.

My daughter and I were on an outing one day. I had spoken with a publisher the day before, and as we were driving in the car, a tear slid down my cheek. Kennedy asked why I was sad. My husband and I have always been real with her and don't hide our struggles. I told her it would take the savings we had planned to use for our future farm to publish this book, and that was a little scary to me. My incredibly sensitive three-year-old said, "Mom, did you know it's okay to be scared?" She was right.

God will do big things with us when we surrender to His plans, especially when we can't see the end result. There are so many times when I've looked around and seen the things I was struggling with as setbacks. What I didn't know was that God had a bigger purpose for those painful moments. In my season of rest, God asked me to set aside my way of doing things. He has a bigger plan, a better way, and a better result if I am willing to set down my way.

YOUR JOURNEY IS UP

Today, I was working in the vegetable trellis, training the vines to go up. They are growing so much on a daily basis. If I don't get out there, they go every which way and get into all kinds of stuff they aren't supposed to. At my house, we talk to our plants and tell them positive things, such as how beautiful they are and how good they are doing. Today, the words that came out of my mouth were, "Remember, your journey is up."

These words hit me like a ton of bricks. This was one of those moments where Jesus was speaking right to me and to you. Remember, your journey is up. Whatever life throws at you, your journey is up. Keep reaching upward. Keep pursuing growth. Keep climbing.

Just look to flowers as your example. Flowers open up their petals, and they depend on their pollinators. This is such a beautiful picture of our dependence on God. If we open our hands and hearts, God will produce fruit!

Go and live empowered. Keep growing and moving forward. Walk in your purpose. Live on purpose, for a purpose. If you are tempted to keep these ideas at arm's length right now, I want to make this personal. I am challenging you to write some of your own next steps right now before you set this book down. Maybe one of them is to go back through the book and engage with the action steps. I sincerely want you to live out your biggest and smallest dreams. Ditch your excuses. Face your fears. Demystify them. Get out your tools and get around whatever obstacles are in your way. I believe you are going to do big things.

I hope that every time you pick up and put down this book, you are inspired to live just a little more empowered. I hope that every time you see it sitting on your bookshelf or coffee table, you are inspired to live empowered. Maybe this book brought out things you didn't even know were in you. Maybe you read something that resonated with who you want to be deep down, but you've been scared or haven't known where to start. This is your time to take action and become the person you want to be.

Get outside of your comfort zone and try some new things. Maybe you read one of the challenges in this book and thought, "That won't make that big of a difference." Try it anyway. Take a chance, be brave, and just try. Keep trying until you become the most confident version of yourself.

This book can be the wind in your sail. It can be your gentle nudge to go live the way you aspire to. It is not about doing things my way but using the ideas and concepts as a starting point and then tweaking them so they suit you. The ideas you put into practice will give you more confidence in how you live.

I tried for so long to live like the happy people in my life did. It took aligning myself with God and living in my deepest values to find the most happiness I have ever had.

God has a big plan for you. You were meant to change the world. Be fearless. I am so excited about your journey. Thank you for sharing a small part of it with me. I am truly honored.

ACKNOWLEDGMENTS

I am thankful for every person on my journey who has encouraged me, invested in me, and believed in me more than I believed in myself. In many ways, you made it possible for me to grow into the person I have become and am still becoming. I almost hesitate to name people because I don't want to miss anyone. Different moments bring different names and faces to mind. There have been critical moments and people who have invested in me for just a snapshot in time but have left a mark that will last forever. There are also people who have invested in me for a season. Then there are those who have invested in me for over a decade. All these people are so valuable in their own way, and each one is shaping and pruning me.

First, my husband Dakota. Thank you for encouraging me to reach for my dreams. There have been so many risks along the way, so thank you for still diving in and believing the best in me.

My precious daughter Kennedy, having you has taught me to defend and fight in a different way than I ever have before. Having you has taught me to have higher standards for myself. Your innocent and unwavering belief is mighty. God has such big plans for you.

To every person who has supported me emotionally and financially through this journey, I am overwhelmed by the way you have shown up in my life. I had built a wall, believing that I had to figure this all out for myself, but you took a sledgehammer to that wall and showed me I am not alone. You did more than support a book—you helped me embrace and be proud of this dream while also tearing down a lie.

I also want to thank my editor, Kelly Flannery. Finding Kelly was divine intervention. She was handpicked by God to do this job, and I have full confidence in her work. I admire her heart, character, and mission to honor God with her work and represent her authors well. She was literally my miracle. I am so thankful for the grace and patience she has had with me through this process and the way she has spoken life and encouragement over it all. You have been a gift to me.

Thank you to every person who has given me a hand up along my journey. This book would not exist without you. To the Hisaws, for taking me under your wing during a vulnerable time and for investing in me for over half my life now. I will be forever grateful for you. Tim Kennedy, for running out of school to catch me when I was having one of my hardest days and for pouring belief over me. Your words in that moment forever changed my life. To Lisa Stabb, who lovingly referred to herself as the surrogate mother to many. Thank you for being a rock in my life. To the Kuulas, who adopted me as a daughter and helped me finish my senior year. Sanne Masters, for hundreds of miles on the road together and for a lifelong friendship. Thank you for going deep, validating my feelings, and searching for the root. Rosan Cowles, for walking through this healing journey with me throughout the years and for walking so close to Jesus His love seeps out of your pores. You are such an encouragement and light. To Pastor Mark Posthuma, who saw my pain when I didn't even know I was hiding from myself. Thank you for being a shelter in the storm and for being part of the hardest and happiest times of my life. To my naturopathic doctor, who has been a huge part of my healing journey. Thank you for being not just a doctor but part of my support system. The tools I have learned from you have changed my life.

To my family, it took me a long time to appreciate the work you did. I see now that you were fighting your own battles. Thank you for fighting. I can only see what I do because I am standing on your shoulders.

BOOK LIST

Wild at Heart	John Eldredge
Captivating	John and Stasi Eldredge
Boundaries	Dr. Henry Cloud and Dr. John Townsend
Boundaries Face to Face	Dr. Henry Cloud and Dr. John Townsend
The Mom Factor	Dr. Henry Cloud and Dr. John Townsend
Sometimes You Win—Sometimes You Learn	John C. Maxwell
Everyone Communicates, Few Connect	John C. Maxwell
Put Your Dream to the Test	John C. Maxwell
Fall in Love, Stay in Love	Willard F. Harley, Jr.
His Needs, Her Needs	Willard F. Harley, Jr.
Wired That Way	Marita Littauer, with insights from Florence Littauer
The One Thing	Gary Keller with Jay Papasan
Start with No	Jim Camp
The 5 Love Languages	Gary Chapman
And Baby Makes Three	John M. Gottman, Ph.D. and Julie Schwartz Gottman, Ph.D.
Parenting With Love and Logic	Foster Cline, M.D. and Jim Fay
Mad About Us	Gary J. Oliver, Ph.D. and Carrie Oliver, M.A.

Your Marriage Masterpiece	Al Janssen
Visioneering	Andy Stanley
Rising Strong	Brené Brown, Ph.D., MSW
The Magic of Thinking Big	David J. Schwartz, Ph.D.
Outliers	Malcolm Gladwell
Finding the Hero in Your Husband, Revisited	Dr. Juli Slattery
The Compound Effect	Darren Hardy
Uninvited	Lysa TerKeurst
The Dream Giver	Bruce Wilkinson
Love & Respect	Dr. Emerson Eggerichs

NOTES